I0786665

Table of Contents

Introduction – Nutrition in 2021

2020 has been an unprecedented, stressful and widely chaotic year for nearly every individual on the planet. When it comes to food and nutrition, national surveys have shown that COVID-19 has directly impacted the eating habits and the nutritional status of many people around the world.

With national stay-at-home orders, people began cooking at home more often and rediscovered the joy (and frustration) of creating homemade sourdough and cooking homemade meals for themselves and their family. For others, closure of gyms and fitness facilities resulted in a surge of home workouts, while others coined the term *"the COVID-19"* referring to a typical weight-gain of 19 pounds as a result of decreased physical activity. Ultimately, the combination of these events over the past year means that health, nutrition and sustainable eating habits are some (of many) issues at the front of minds of individuals.

Now, in 2021, the interest in nutrition and healthy eating has not plateaued but continues to surge as new research emerges demonstrating the importance of underlying metabolic health and its relationship to health and disease. As diet is the second greatest behaviour risk for developing chronic diseases (after smoking), undesirable changes in diet can put more individuals at risk of developing chronic diseases in the future.

The good news? Granted sufficient access to food, it is in our power to change our dietary habits for the better. However, with the rise of scientific misinformation, including unverified blog posts, anecdotal stories or social media posts by who knows what, it can be confusing to know what the best way is to eat. Different healthy eating, diet and nutritional advice is everywhere and is often contradicting. Food can be complicated, and **it's because we do not simply eat to fulfill the biological requirements of the human body.**

While food provides energy and nutrients, it also provides a source of culture, a sense of belonging, a reason to gather and socialize, and a source of delicious, fulfilling pleasure. From a scientific point of view, our biology supports these associations as our appetite is regulated by not one, but two systems: physiological hunger and hedonic hunger.

Physiological hunger occurs in the presence of simply not eating enough food, where signals from our brain and our digestive system will produce the signs and symptoms associated with hunger to ensure food intake is on the horizon to survive.

However, even when calorie and nutrient needs are met **hedonic hunger** can override physiological signals. This means that the associations we make between food and pleasure, such as a chocolate cake, can interfere with physiological signals of fullness allowing us to overeat.

Ultimately, the overlapping of these pathways is another reason why we have a complicated relationship with food, strengthening the notion that we are not simply wired to consume food solely to replenish our energy and nutrient needs.

Is there one optimal, one-size fits all approach to eating? In short, the answer is no. Science consistently shows that there is not one best diet for human consumption, but there are certainly healthful foods that contribute to an overall healthy dietary pattern.

This means that in this book, you will learn the basics of nutrition science based on the most recent research to ensure that you have the knowledge you need to make better dietary decisions, for good, in 2021.

Let's get started.

Chapter 1: Nutrition Basics – Carbohydrates, Protein and Fat

In this chapter, we will go over the building blocks of nutrition known as the macronutrients. Our body gets energy from three main macronutrients: carbohydrates, protein and fat, where each plays an important role in our body.

You may have heard of someone counting their "macros". This is short for macronutrients, and includes the amount of carbohydrates, fat and protein they are consuming each day. Carbohydrates and proteins contain 4 calories per gram, while fat contains 9 calories per gram.

There is a lot of debate about what ratio of macronutrients is optimal for human health, however science suggests that there is not one optimal ratio. Therefore, in this chapter we will go over all the most up to date basics of nutritional science about these macronutrients, so you are empowered with the knowledge to make your own decisions.

Carbohydrates

The carbohydrate is a cyclic organic molecule consisting of six carbon elements. Each of these carbohydrates have a water molecule attached to them, thus bearing the name, carbohydrates. Each gram of carbohydrates provides 4 calories of energy.

Carbohydrates, which are found in many different foods. Ranging from sweet, sugary desserts to whole grain pasta, sweet potatoes, legumes and even maple-syrup. However, carbohydrates **are** the subject of much debate. Should we eat low carbohydrates? What are complex carbohydrates? Is the fructose in fruit bad for you? What about the keto diet and diabetes?

Rather than giving one definitive answer, which is almost entirely impossible as **nutritional science consistently shows that there is not one single best diet for human consumption,** we will cover the basics of carbohydrate nutrition: including the primary sources of carbohydrates, how carbohydrates are digested and debunking some common myths about this macronutrient that you likely already had for breakfast.

What are the primary sources of carbohydrates?

The word carbohydrates may bring about warm memories of fresh baked breads, delicate pastries and rich, creamy pastas. For others, they may think of sweet-potato fries, their favourite potato chips and ice-cream. Others may be even more adventurous in their definition, dreaming up lentils and chickpeas, carrots, potatoes, turnips and fruits such as bananas, apples, strawberries and mangoes.

All of food items above contain primarily the carbohydrate macronutrient, and in varying amounts and of varying complexities.

A food being high in carbohydrates is not always equitable to being high in sugar. Carbohydrates is the umbrella terms for all the different hydrated carbons. And when we differentiate between digestible and non-digestible, we can understand our net carbohydrate intake.

Our net carbohydrate intake considers the amount of **digestible carbohydrates** that we are consuming. Digestible carbohydrates include sugars and starches, while indigestible carbohydrates include fibres and sugar alcohols. On a nutrition label, the number of sugars and starched are included under "total carbohydrates". This means you can calculate your net carbohydrate intake using the following formula:

Net carbohydrates = [Total Carbohydrates — (Fibres + Sugar Alcohols])

Complex carbohydrates are higher in fibre, meaning that they have less net, or digestible, carbohydrates. When we digest a complex carbohydrate, it will take longer to release the individual molecules of sugars, and the fibres will slow down our digestion, increase satiety and allow a slower release of sugar into our bloodstream. Complex carbohydrates, such as whole grains and legumes, also contain protein which will further activate our satiety signals, such as the PPY hormone.

Fun Fact: Have you ever heard about fibre lowering cholesterol levels? It's true! Bile acids contain cholesterol, where insoluble fibre will bind to bile acids and will be excreted instead of reabsorbed back into the body.

In contrast, simple carbohydrates don't need any breakdown of starch, and contains no fibre. Therefore, as it states in its name, the carbohydrate is absorbed simply as sugar and ready to be used as energy when it enters the bloodstream.

How are carbohydrates digested?

The digestion of carbohydrates begins with enzymes in our saliva and will continue to breakdown with the acidity of our stomach fluids. After the mixture is turned and churned into our stomach, it's pH will neutralize as it passes into the small intestine, where most of the absorption into the bloodstream will occur. The carbohydrate will be absorbed as singular sugars—monosaccharides including glucose and fructose.

Fun fact: Simple table sugar is composed of the disaccharide, sucrose which is 50% glucose and 50% fructose. It will be absorbed into the bloodstream as these individual components.

When there is an increase in glucose, our pancreas will release the hormone insulin, which allows our insulin-dependent organs, such as muscle, heart and fat tissue to access glucose for energy.

Is the sugar in fruit bad for you?

Fruits contain naturally occurring fructose and glucose carbohydrates.

Let's contrast glucose with fructose for a moment. Glucose will elicit a release of insulin, however fructose does not. But the latter is more associated with weight-gain, insulin-resistance and metabolic syndrome.

In order to be used for energy, fructose must be metabolized in the liver first, where it will become glucose, free fatty acids or lactate. This will increase blood glucose, and then allow for insulin signalling. Metabolic and oxidative stress can occur when **large amounts of fructose** are consumed—which occurs when it is consumed in large quantities, such as is soft-drinks and processed sweet desserts.

This means that the small amount of naturally occurring fructose in fruits is perfectly fine. Also remember that fruit comes with other types of carbohydrates—starch and fibres, and therefore is **not associated** with the same metabolic concerns as consuming high-fructose corn-syrup.

The bottom line? Skip the soft drinks but have the all the fruit with breakfast.

Does insulin make you gain weight?

In normal physiology, it does not.

Our insulin is tightly regulated when we have normal insulin signalling, and as long as we aren't consuming an excess of energy, insulin will not have any excess energy to store as fat.

This changes when we have insulin resistance, where our bodies compensate by pumping out more insulin to get the same amount of blood sugar down to normal. The hyperinsulinemia in this context can cause weight-gain.

But do carbs make you gain weight?

The issue is that weight-gain arises when we consume an energy surplus of any macronutrient, including fats, protein or carbohydrate.

Once insulin has fulfilled its duty in dispersing nutrients to where they need to be, any extra energy will be rearranged into a triglyceride to be put into fat storage. This fat storage around our organs will make insulin-signalling more difficult, causing hyperinsulinemia and weight-gain.

What's the hype with low-carb diets and diabetes?

Contrary to popular belief, the low-carbohydrate diet can be traced back to centuries ago, and it is far from being a new discovery within the world of food, diet and nutrition.

In what is known as the "*pre-insulin*" era, researchers and physicians scoured out different dietary interventions which would alleviate the "sweet urine" of those with diabetes.

As early as 1706, John Rollo, a Surgeon-General <u>successfully treated a patient by dietary restriction</u>—achieving a similar pathophysiological response as a carbohydrate-restricted diet. These ideas propagated throughout history, where low-carbohydrate, sugar-free and even "starvation" diets were the mainstay nutritional intervention of those with diabetes mellitus.

Fun Fact: Type II diabetes is caused by defective insulin signalling-inhibiting our body's ability to access the glucose energy in our bloodstream, causing high-blood sugar. The insulin resistance is caused by the excess of fat deposits around organs and it's ensuing systemic inflammatory response. Type I diabetes is an auto-immune disease targeting the insulin-producing beta-cells of our pancreas, rendering them non-functional.

After the isolation and official discovery of insulin by Canadian cardiologist, Frederick Banting, in 1921, the peptide-hormone went almost immediately to pharmaceutical production to begin relieving people for the very first time, of their once unresolvable diabetes.

Insulin led way to a new course of life for those with diabetes. They could now mimic the normal physiological state of their metabolism, meaning they could skip the starvation or low-carbohydrate diets and could now enjoy their carbohydrates as long as they titrated accordingly with their insulin medication. The insulin medication also improved their co-morbidity outlook, reducing nerve damage, blindness and cardiovascular disease risk.

What's the difference between a low-carb and ketogenic diet?

On a ketogenic diet, we alter our macronutrient proportions to high fat, moderate-low protein and very-low carbohydrates. In doing this, we deplete our glycogens store and tap into our fat stores to derive energy, essentially simulating the same physiological response during starvation. To reach ketosis, we need to keep our net carbohydrate intake usually under 50 g, which would roughly be the equivalent of 2 medium fruits or 1 cup of rice.

When people with diabetes embark on these low-carbohydrate diets, they are essentially going back in time to the early nutritional interventions of diabetes (primarily Type I), namely the "starvation" or low-carbohydrate diets which were prescribed by the physicians of the 18th century.

Is low carbohydrate the answer for resolving type II diabetes?

Could reverting back to the low-carbohydrate diet be the ideal way to nutritionally intervene with a person with type II diabetes?

Potentially, but the diet is not yet considered to have strong-enough evidence, therefore clinicians are often hesitant to incorporate into their practice. Also let's remember that diabetes is much more complex than restricting an individual macronutrient.

If a decision is made to go on a ketogenic diet, it is strongly recommended to consult with a Registered Dietitian to understand the diet within the complexity of diabetes. They can help you navigate several considerations to individualize the diet to your needs.

For example, …. *Will you be reducing your hypoglycemic medications? What are your lipid levels and cardiovascular disease risk? Are you an athlete? Are you pregnant? Can you afford the diet? Which recipes will suit the diet and your nutrient needs?*

These are important considerations to make when altering your diet drastically.

Should I go low carbohydrate to lose weight?

Remember, low-carbohydrate diets will deplete your glycogen stores primarily found in the liver and muscles. Glycogen, the storage form of carbohydrates, is stored alongside with water—*therefore, much of the initial rapid weight-loss observed is attributed to the water lost alongside the glycogen.*

A <u>recent RCT</u> (n=600) examined the long-term weight loss of those consuming isocaloric deficits of high-fat, low-carb and low-fat, high-carb diets. While the low-carb group lost the most initial weight (due to depleted glycogen stores), the total weight loss amongst both groups remained the same in the long-term.

Therefore—**the best diet for weight-loss is one that you can stick to**, and nutritional science consistently shows that there is not one best diet for weight-loss.

We cannot crown one diet king and prescribe this to a population—the human body is too complex and specific to each individual. For you, achieving a calorie deficit may be easier on a lower-carbohydrate diet, for others they may feel more satiated incorporating complex carbohydrates.

Which carbohydrates should I focus on to stay healthy?

Focus on complex carbohydrates, which will have a source of soluble and/or insoluble fibre which can help you feel fuller, improve glycemic levels and help reduce cholesterol levels.

Good sources of complex carbohydrates include:

- Whole grain breads, oatmeal and quinoa.
- Sweet potatoes, broccoli and carrots.
- Legumes, such as chickpeas, lentils and beans.
- Fruits, such as apples, bananas and berries.

The most concerning carbohydrate to avoid are items containing *high-fructose corn syrup*, which is found in sweetened beverages, breakfast cereals and many processed foods—this fructose-based sweetener has been shown to induce insulin resistance, even when it is not consumed within an excess of energy needs.

A sweet, last word.

In the world of confusing nutritional science and never-ending fad diets, simply breaking down what a carbohydrate actually is can bring us to a somewhat relieving conclusion—*if we don't want to, we don't need to cut out all carbohydrates.*

On the other hand, if we think a low-carbohydrate approach might help us in terms of weight loss or disease management, *a Registered Dietitian can help us manage the risk-benefit ratio of doing so.*

It's tempting to delve into the next fad diet in pursuit of the hyped-up health benefits, anecdotal success stories and drastic weight loss based on limited evidence—however let's consider this: **The rise of obesity and type II diabetes is not because somewhere along the way, we stopped consuming a low-carbohydrate diet.**

Instead, let's work to find a way of eating which is sustainable to us—a way of eating which doesn't focus on the singularity of one macronutrient over another—and rather considers our nutritional goals, lifestyle, cooking skills, current disease management and quality of life.

Protein

Where can we get protein? The truth is a lot of places. Chickpeas, tofu, eggs, Greek yogurt, lentils, nuts, chicken, beef, fish and liver – just to name a few. For you, it might be a bit different, including more or less animal-or plant-based sources. The similarity between most people, however, is that we are **likely already consuming enough protein**.

In 2021, "*high protein*" is expected to continue as a potent nutritional buzzword, as it was in 2020. From gracing sugary cereal boxes to enticing your green smoothie with a $1.50 add-in, the media and food industry makes it seem as if we can never get enough of this macronutrient.

So, what exactly is the hype about protein? Do we really need more protein than before? Should we take BCAA's? What types of plant-based proteins are the best? What the heck even is protein?

Similar to the chapter about **carbohydrates,** this chapter will delve into the basics, common questions and misconceptions surrounding protein, delivered in an unbiased and evidence-based approach—because nutritional science consistently shows us that there is no single best diet for human consumption.

Are amino acids only the building blocks of muscle protein?

When we think of amino acids, we traditionally know them as the building blocks of muscle protein. While this is intuitive, and mostly true, the reasons for ensuring you meet all your essential amino acids goes beyond simply building muscle.

Amino acids are chains of carbon, with an ammonia group and a carboxylic acid group. Strictly dietary speaking, the most important type of amino acids are **essential amino acids.**

As humans, we lack the enzymatic machinery to synthesize 9 out of the 20 amino acids to meet our body's needs. Therefore, we must acquire these amino acids through diet. A way to remember this is that essential amino acids are "essential" to obtain through diet.

Fun Fact: The nine essential amino acids are valine, phenylalanine, histidine, lysine, methionine, tryptophan, isoleucine, threonine and leucine.

Once the protein we eat is digested into amino acids, they can be used for energy, protein synthesis, or other biosynthesis pathways.

This means that **amino acids are not only the building blocks of muscle-protein.**

What are the other functions of amino acids?

Amino acids can be <u>metabolized into neurotransmitters,</u> such as **serotonin** from tryptophan. Serotonin is our "feel-good" neurotransmitter and can also regulate our intestinal movement. The amino acid is converted into serotonin primarily in our gut microbiome. We will talk more about serotonin in the chapter on mental health and nutrition.

There are numerous other examples of other uses of amino acids. **Epinephrine** is derived from tyrosine and helps us activate our fight-or-flight response. **Creatine** is synthesized from three amino acids: glycine, arginine and methionine and supplies ATP energy molecules to our muscles. **Histamine** is derived from histidine and is released during an allergic reaction.

Similarly, combinations of different strands of amino acids to create protein is **not solely destined for protein found in our muscles**.

Protein synthesis can also include enzymes, transport proteins, and hemoglobin, which is a carrier for oxygen molecules in our red-blood cells. In fact, a deficiency in histidine (an essential amino acid) will disrupt the protein synthesis of hemoglobin, <u>potentially resulting in anemia</u>.

How does protein and branched chain amino acids stimulate muscle-protein synthesis?

Muscle-protein synthesis (MPS) is stimulated by the ingestion of essential amino acids. <u>Strong research</u> has consistently shown that the essential amino- acid **leucine** plays a key role in stimulating MPS, especially after performing resistance training. MPS is stimulated when leucine activates mTORC1, a receptor in our cells which is responsible for nutrient metabolism, including protein synthesis.

Leucine is a **branched-chain amino acid** (BCAA), which refers to its chemical structure. Isoleucine and valine are also BCAA's, and all BCAA's are essential amino acids. Knowing that BCAA's stimulate MPS, sport nutrition supplement companies have been quick to market *"BCAA supplements"* to enhance MPS.

However, BCAAs appear to work best when they are **consumed alongside other essential-amino acids.** In fact, one study showed that solely consuming BCAA's results in stimulating 50% less MPS compared to 100% whey protein.

The bottom line? BCAA supplements are not required for stimulating MPS. A complete source of protein, including whole foods, is best for stimulating MPS.

Why can't I simply eat more protein to build more muscle?

We know that essential amino acids, including BCAA's, stimulate MPS, but how could it be **increased**? Unfortunately, simply eating more protein, even if it has an optimal amino acid profile will not increase MPS.

We need to create a reason for our muscles to synthesize more protein, which can be achieved through stressing our muscles in a new workout regime (*especially resistance training*), encountering a sickness or injury (*although not recommended*) and the normal growth experienced in children.

Furthermore, protein has **no official storage space** in our body. Unlike carbohydrates which are stored as glycogen and fat which is stored away in adipose tissue, extra dietary protein does not equate to extra protein synthesis "stored" into our muscles. Instead, it can cause weight-gain as the extra carbon-backbones are converted into triglycerides for fat storage.

Not convinced that our muscles don't store protein. Think of it this way. Our muscles serve many functions: strength, stability, immune function and even heat. Therefore, tapping into our muscles for protein and energy compromises functionality. This may happen under periods of starvation or increased protein needs and inadequate intake, such as after surgery.

Knowing all this, how can I ensure my diet covers all essential amino acid and protein needs?

While the nutritional science may seem overwhelming and sometimes confusing, the bottom line concerning adequate protein intake while achieving an optimal amino acid profile is quite simple: ***Eat a variety of protein containing foods.***

Foods with a complete amino acid profile can include **both** animal and plant sources of protein. Notably, quinoa and soy are complete sources of plant-based proteins, however amino-acid digestibility of these foods may be decreased due to fibre and other non-nutritional components.

If you are seeking a nutritional supplement, such as in the form of a protein powder, ensure it contains **all essential amino acids** and ideally at least 2.7 g of leucine per serving. Supplements containing **whey** or **pea** protein isolates may be the best choice due to their complete essential amino acid profiles, and high leucine content.

Remember that whole protein foods also contain BCAA's. For example, 100g of chicken contains approximately 8 g of BCAAs, while 1/2 cup of Greek yogurt will provide 5 g.

Fun Fact: Why are complete proteins so important? Protein synthesis can be thought of as an "all-or-nothing" process. Even if we lack 1% of the amino acids required, the remaining 99% amino acids present will be degraded, and the protein will not be synthesized.

A strong, bottom line.

While protein nutritional jargon is fed to us by the spoonful these days, it is reassuring to know that most healthy individuals can meet their protein needs through whole foods, such as the protein sources described above.

Also, remember that the best diet for you is one that is sustainable. This year, instead of focusing on the singularity of one macronutrient over another—consider your nutritional goals, lifestyle, cooking skills, current disease management and quality of life.

Fat

Let's imagine it's 2005. You're strolling through the yogurt aisle at your local grocery store supermarket. Between switching songs on your iPod Nano and chatting on your new Motorola cellphone, you are haphazardly comparing labels between yogurts. Instantaneously, you toss the one with the *"fat-free"* label into your cart. Because the fat we eat is that fat we wear, right?

Fast-forward sixteen years later to 2021, and we find people with exact opposite attitude's when it comes to fat. **Fat is everywhere** and is regarded by some as the macronutrient which might finally save us from ourselves. They say, "This time the butter, bacon and coconut oil will finally reverse complex chronic diseases, like diabetes and obesity!".

The battle between the high-fat and low-fat philosophies has left a sour aftertaste of confusion, before we even finish our plate. *Is coconut oil healthy? What about saturated fat? Which fats are essential? Should I follow a high-fat diet, such as the ketogenic diet?*

Developing a base in nutritional science could help people tease out some basic fact from fiction. Since nutritional science shows that **there is not one single best diet for human consumption**, this chapter will delve into the **nutritional basics of fat** so you can better digest the next nutrition hype headline you come across.

Fat Physiology

First of all—we can store a lot of energy as fat.

Remember the infamous "*oil and vinegar*" doesn't mix science experiment? This property of fat actually comes in handy physiologically and is the reason why fat (or triglycerides) is our preferred **stored** source of energy. One gram of fat contains 9 calories, over twice as much energy as carbohydrates and protein.

Adipose tissue is estimated to store up to **100,000 calories of energy, whereas glycogen only stores about 2,000 calories of energy**

If we think in terms of basic physics, fat holds a lot more *potential energy* compared to glycogen stores. Glycogen, or the storage form of glucose from carbohydrates must be stored with "bulky" water, and <u>only provides enough energy to last about a day</u> (about 2,000 calories worth of stored energy).

On the other hand, triglyceride stores in our adipose tissue is estimated to store up to <u>100,000 calories as fat</u>. This is why we are able to survive in prolonged periods of fasting. We can tap into our adipose tissue, transforming triglycerides to form ketone bodies for energy utilization. This is also part of the physiology behind those following ketogenic or fasting diets.

The Healthy Fats

Omega-3 and Omega-6 Fatty Acids

The only essential fats for the human body are the two polyunsaturated fats, **omega-3** and **omega-6 fatty acids.** Polyunsaturated refers to the fatty acids carbon structure having more than one double bond.

This means that fats such as omega 9s, saturated fats and cholesterol are *not* essential nutrients. Our body can make enough of these nutrients itself without obtaining extra from our diet.

Omega-3 fatty acids are found in foods such as fatty-fish, walnuts, chia, flaxseed and their oils. These fatty acids play a role in anti-inflammatory processes and brain and cognitive development. On the other hand, consuming large amounts of omega-6 fatty acids, such as in sunflower and soybean oil are associated with inflammation.

As inflammation is the basis of many diseases, including metabolic syndrome, the general principal is to ensure that the ratio of your omega-3 fatty acid intake is *higher* than your omega-6 fatty acid intake. This is because both fatty acids compete for the same enzymes within the body.

What's the difference between omega-3, ALA, DHA and EPA?

As mentioned above, omega-3 is a polyunsaturated fatty acid, or a PUFA. All this means is that these fats have one more bond on its carbon chain compared to monounsaturated fats. There are three types of omega-3 fatty acids, known as ALA, DHA and EPA.

However, ALA, DHA and EPA are all synthesized from the same omega-3 fatty acid. You can think of the omega-3 fatty acid as a starting point, and once digested in our body it will be converted by our enzymes into ALA, DHA and EPA, and in that order. These omega-3 fatty acids are essential for **brain and cognitive development**, especially in neurodevelopment of children, teens and in-utero for pregnant mothers.

If we are following primarily a plant-based or vegan diet, we are likely sourcing ALA omega-3 fatty acids from walnuts, chia seeds, flax seeds and their oils. ALA will be converted by enzymes in our body into EPA and DHA.

On the other hand, when we consume foods such as fatty fish and fortified eggs, we are sourcing EPA and DHA straight from the source, meaning it doesn't have to go through the rather inefficient enzymatic process.

Are plant or animal sources of omega-3 better?

As mentioned above, plant-based sources of omega-3 fatty acids, such as flax seed, chia seed, walnuts and their oils are most commonly found in the **ALA** form and will be converted in our body to DHA and EPA.

However, one downside to consuming plant-based sources of omega-3 fatty acids is that they are less efficiently used in the body. Remember that the end goal is to produce DHA and EPA from ALA. In humans, our body can only convert 1-15% of plant-based ALA into these needed end-products.

Therefore, for those following a strict vegan diet may consider supplementing with DHA and EPA. They can be found as micro-algae supplements.

Also, those who are pregnant, or who live with diabetes may have a decreased conversion efficiency and could benefit from consuming EPA and DHA from the source or consuming a plant-based micro-algae supplementation.

On the other hand, we can obtain DHA and EPA straight from the source by consuming animal-based foods such as fatty fish and eggs. Consuming two servings of fatty fish is enough to meet your DHA and EPA requirement.

The bottom line is that it can be difficult to get enough DPA and EPA if you are vegan, pregnant or living with diabetes. For these populations, speak with your doctor or dietitian about supplementing. If you regularly consume fish and eggs, you should be fine without a supplement.

Olive Oil, Nuts, Seeds & Avocado

Now that we have covered polyunsaturated fats, lets dive into monounsaturated fats. Olive oil, nuts, seeds & avocado are monounsaturated fats, which refers to its single double bond on its carbon structure. These fats have numerous health benefits.

The infamous <u>PREDI-MED</u> study found a significant reduction in cardiovascular disease risk when individuals supplemented their diet with extra nuts and olive oil compared to the control, low-fat group. An important consideration in this study is that they were supplementing on-top of a healthy, Mediterranean style diet.

This suggests that olive-oil & nuts have a *synergistic effect* of when combined with a diet rich in fruits & vegetables, whole grains and low in saturated & trans-fat. In other words, the health benefits of these foods come from the context of the diet they are added onto, and cannot be achieved by adding copious amounts of olive oil and nuts to an unhealthy diet

Nuts & seeds are not only a source of good fat and protein but are also a good source of **arginine**, an amino acid which is a precursor to nitric oxide. Nitric oxide is a chemical which helps promote blood flow and prevent heart attacks. They also contains soluble fibre, and other phytochemicals which help lower LDL-cholesterol and increase HDL cholesterol.

The bottom line is that to reap these health benefits, add a few extra servings of nuts and olive oil on top of an existing healthy diet, rich in fruits, vegetables, legumes, whole grains and lean proteins.

The Not-So Healthy Fats

We've gone over the good fats, including the polyunsaturated and the monounsaturated fats – but now what about the not-so-healthy fats? In this section, we will discuss saturated and trans-fats and their implication for health.

What's the difference between saturated and trans-fats?

Saturated fats are often naturally occurring and are found in both animal and plant foods. On the other hand, trans-fats (*with the exception of some dairy products*) are not naturally occurring and are the by-product of food process known as hydrogenation to make a product more shelf-stable or solid, such as butter, margarine and many processed junk foods.

The negative impacts of trans-fats on health are indisputable. Found primarily in commercially prepared foods such as chips, cakes, pastries and sweets, the fatty acids resulting from food processing have led to national-public health campaigns banning the nutrient.

On the other hand, saturated fats are officially recommended to be limited <10% of total energy intake, mostly due to their role in increasing LDL-cholesterol, a risk factor for cardiovascular disease. But exceptions and confusion exist around saturated fat as there are *many different types of saturated fatty acid*s—all with slightly different impact on our health.

However, the bottom line on saturated fat remains that reductions in cardiovascular disease risk are seen when saturated fats are replaced with other fats. This refers to the omega-3 fatty acids, monounsaturated and polyunsaturated fatty acids discussed above.

Should I limit meat since it is high in saturated fat?

Let's go back to the PREDI-MED study, where heart healthy benefits were observed in individuals who consumed animal meats while following a healthy Mediterranean style diet.

Within this context, consuming animal meats for protein in a Mediterranean diet-pattern rich in antioxidant containing fruits and vegetables, omega-3 fatty acids and fibre-containing whole grains, is *definitely* health promoting.

On the other hand, if the mainstays of your meals are solely red meat and fried chicken, you may want to consider limiting your intake of meat and replacing it with healthier sources of fat and plant-based proteins. This is because excess amounts of animal saturated fat can raise LDL-cholesterol levels, which is a risk factor for cardiovascular disease.

Are plant-based sources of saturated fat, such as coconut oil healthy?

Coconut oil is a notorious plant-based source of saturated fat, which was hugely successful in captivating the North American market. In fact, the global market for coconut oil is estimated to reach <u>$4.9 billion by 2024</u>.

Coconut oil is a type of medium-chain triglyceride (MCT), made up primarily of lauric acid. Its chemical structure allows it to be metabolized directly in the liver for energy. <u>MCTs are also not stored in adipose tissue</u>, and are rather used for energy compared to long-chain fatty acids. This means that instead of being stored as fat, they will be used up quickly by our body for energy.

Coconut oil has been seen to <u>raise both LDL and HDL-cholesterol levels</u>. LDL cholesterol is known as "bad" cholesterol and HDL cholesterol is known as "good cholesterol".

 However, the studies revealed that coconut oil raised the bad, LDL-cholesterol to a <u>much greater extent</u> which poses a risk factor for cardiovascular disease. Therefore, it is not recommended to use coconut oil, and should be replaced with healthy fats such as omega-3s, monounsaturated and polyunsaturated fat.

What is MCT oil?

With the craze around coconut oil, many food manufacturers have turned to start producing medium chain triglyceride (MCT) oil to get in on the hype. You may have seen MCT oil advertised as a mix-ins for your smoothies, coffees and even as a stand-alone supplement. But is there enough evidence to supports its use? Let's dive in.

Medium-chain triglycerides found in the form of caprylic acid, a type of saturated fat, is primarily used in commercial MCT oils. Historically, MCT oil been used for those with fat absorption issues. The oil requires less enzymes to breakdown the fat in our digestive tract, allowing it to become more easily absorbed into our blood stream.

Once this easy-to-absorb fat is circulating in our blood, it will travel directly to our liver to be converted into a source of energy known as a **ketone body**. Our body can run on one of two fuel sources: sugar from carbohydrates or ketone bodies from fat. Under normal circumstances, our body thrives on sugar as fuel and will only use ketone bodies if we are starving, consuming a low-carbohydrate diet or during intense exercise. This is known as ketosis.

If ketosis is brought on by a low-carbohydrate diet, there has been reported health benefits including weight-loss and fat loss as our body burns our own fat stores for a source of energy. However, consuming more fat, such as through an MCT oil supplement **will not bring on the same health benefits as ketosis unless if we are following a low-carbohydrate diet at the same time**.

The bottom line is that while MCT oil can be helpful for those who have trouble digesting fat and will be converted into ketone bodies for energy, it will not provide the same health benefits associated with ketone bodies production in ketosis.

Is the saturated fat in dairy, such as milk, cheese and yogurt healthy?

Different from the saturated fat found in coconut oil and red meat, saturated fat found in dairy products, such as milk, yogurt and cheese have actually been found to have a **neutral impact** on bad cholesterol, or LDL-cholesterol.

This is because while the saturated fats from dairy products elevate LDL-cholesterol, they also **increase the size** of the LDL particle. What makes LDL-cholesterol dangerous is not the cholesterol itself, but it's small size which is convenient for slipping into blood vessels causing inflammation. Therefore, increasing the size of the LDL-particle through dairy consumption decreases these risks.

However, dairy products are usually consumed as source of **protein**, and not fat. It's good to know that it's saturated fat is not seen to adversely affect heart health, but we should still source omega-3, monounsaturated and polyunsaturated fatty acids elsewhere within the diet.

Does eating too much cholesterol raise my cholesterol levels?

It is a myth that the cholesterol we consume in our diet influences the cholesterol levels in our blood. Did you notice that above we only spoke about saturated fat influencing cholesterol levels? That's right, the dietary cholesterol we consume, found in animal foods, <u>does not raise blood cholesterol levels</u>. Blood cholesterol levels are more related to the amount of saturated fat we consume.

You might start to put the two and two together: isn't a lot of saturated fat found in cholesterol containing animal foods, such as beef, butter and cheese? Yes, and knowing this can help us better evaluate and choose healthier animal-based foods.

For example, animal-based foods such as shrimp and eggs are high in cholesterol but **lower in saturated fat**, which can avoid spiking LDL cholesterol. Replacing saturated fat with omega-3 fatty acids, fibres, monounsaturated and polyunsaturated fatty acids can also help reduce LDL-cholesterol and reduce cardiovascular disease risks.

What is the difference between good and bad cholesterol?

The "bad" carrier of cholesterol is known as LDL, or low-density lipoprotein. The "good" carrier of cholesterol is known as HDL, or high-density lipoprotein.

Under normal conditions, our liver tightly regulates the amount of LDL found in our bloodstream to keep us healthy.

However, this regulation can be disrupted by *too much dietary saturated fat* or genetic conditions causing too much production of cholesterol and not enough uptake into our liver.

When we have too much LDL in our blood, it becomes prone to oxidation, slips into the lining of our blood vessels and promotes atherosclerosis, or the thickening of blood vessels which can cause heart attacks.

On the other hand, HDL can actually *decrease* the amount of LDL in circulation which is known through a pathway called "reverse cholesterol transport". It regulates the amount of LDL and is the reason why HDL cholesterol is known as "good cholesterol".

How do my food choices influence my blood test results?

Has your doctor ever told you that your cholesterol or triglyceride levels are too high? The truth is that our fat and carbohydrate intake are reflected in our bloodstream.

Therefore, it's not as simple as blaming "fat" or "carbs" on sup-optimal blood test results. It ultimately depends on the type of fat or carbohydrates, and the overall context of our usual diet.

For example:

1) Refined carbohydrates (think cakes, cookies, white bread, pasta, soda) and alcohol will **increase triglycerides** and **reduce HDL-cholesterol**.

2) Complex carbohydrates, such as fruits, vegetables, whole grains, legumes and polyunsaturated fat, such as omega-3 fatty acids will **decrease LDL-cholesterol.**

3) Saturated fat intake, such as from red meat, coconut oil and processed foods will **decrease triglycerides** but increase **LDL-cholesterol**

The bottom-line

Ensuring that your diet has **at least 20% of calories coming from fat**.

Healthy sources of fat primarily consist of omega-3, polyunsaturated and monounsaturated fats—all which have positive cardiovascular disease outcomes when *replacing* the saturated or trans-fat in our diet.

Enjoy healthy sources of fats, including:

- Fatty fish, such as salmon (*Best source of essential omega-3 fatty acids*)
- Extra-virgin olive oil
- Avocado
- Nuts, seeds & their butters

Remember—there is not one macronutrient, including fat, which is the gatekeeper of health, longevity and optimal nutrition. Instead, focus on the **totality of your diet** which encompasses healthful choices surrounding fat, carbohydrate and protein alike.

Chapter 2: Sports Nutrition & Fitness

Now that we have covered the basics of the macronutrients: carbohydrates, protein and fat let challenge our knowledge with a real-world application of these macronutrients: sports nutrition & optimizing athletic performance.

Nutritional supplements to enhance athletic performance have been used as early as 400–500 B.C, where athletes and warriors are thought to have ate foods such as <u>deer liver and lion heart</u> to improve strength and bravery.

Nowadays, our greater scientific understanding of physiology and metabolism has allowed us to produce a global sports nutrition market valued at over <u>50 billion dollars USD</u>.

Even the widely popular ketogenic diet has made its way into the sports nutrition world, where athletes can *"up-regulate"* fat-oxidation enzymes and improve training outcomes.

But does this mean that you should do it to?

It depends, because **nutrition is highly nuanced**, and even more when it is applied to sports and exercise, as everyone's metabolism, gene expression, fitness level and medical history is different. Therefore, this chapter on sports nutrition will serve as a *"crash course"* for covering the basics of sports nutrition, including:

- **Difference between aerobic and anaerobic metabolism**
- **Water**
- **Carbohydrates**
- **Protein and Protein Supplementation**
- **Fat and Low-Carb Ketogenic Diets, or "Training Low"**
- **Branched-Chain Amino Acids, Creatine, and Antioxidant Supplementation**

Aerobic and anaerobic metabolism in exercise

These are the two main types of metabolisms which occur during exercise. Knowing these will help us understand the types of nutrients our body prefers as fuel during different types of exercise.

First, **aerobic metabolism** refers to what's going on in the cells of our body when there is oxygen available. This is our metabolism during most endurance exercises, such as biking, swimming and jogging.

Most sports are also considered endurance exercise. During aerobic metabolism, oxygen is available to our cells to use carbohydrate, fat or protein for energy. Most of the time, our body will prefer to utilize our **fat stores** during endurance exercise.

In **anaerobic metabolism**, there is little or no oxygen available to our muscle cells. This happens during strength-training, such as weightlifting, high-intensity-interval training (HITT) and fast-sprints.

When there is less oxygen available, our body can only use **carbohydrates** from **glycogen storage** through the anaerobic lactic acid-cycle, which is why we get a build-up of lactic-acid during these kinds of exercises.

Remembering the differences between these two exercises will help us later on in this chapter.

Hydration is Key

Water is the original nutritional "*supplement*", since the heat our muscles creates during exercise causes us to lose water.

Dehydration during exercise can reduce strength, endurance, mental focus and recovery. In fact, we can lose up to 0.5–2L of water per hour which can push many athletes to drink as much water as possible.

However, over-hydration is also a concern during exercise. *Hyponatremia*, or low sodium in our blood can result as a consequence of drinking too much water in combination of the salt lost through our sweat. This can be even more dangerous than dehydration.

A sports drink containing sodium, electrolytes and carbohydrates may be beneficial during exercises which cause lots of sweating, or if the exercise is >2 hours.

Following our thirst cues and drinking at regular intervals is usually enough to cover our hydration needs before, during and after exercise. During exercise, **400–800 ml of water/hour** is thought to be adequate.

Carbohydrates

Carbohydrates are the preferred source of energy for our muscles during high-intensity, **anaerobic exercise.** *Why?* Because basic high-school biochemistry, and solid scientific evidence says so.

First of all, carbohydrates have the advantage of **generating more ATP** (*the energy currency of our cells*) for our muscle cells per volume of oxygen, compared to protein or fat. The greater intensity of exercise we perform, the harder we breathe (less oxygen available). Therefore, our body goes for the path of least resistance, oxidizing glucose into lactic acid for muscle energy.

When we exhaust our muscle and liver glycogen stores, it is often referred to as *"hitting the wall"*, resulting in fatigue.

Therefore, **maximal glycogen storage** is a key consideration in all stages of sport nutrition.

How many carbs should I eat before, during and after exercise?

Carbohydrate requirements vary drastically by the individual, but in general athletes require **5–7 g/kg/day**. Athletes can mix and match the following strategies to meet their carbohydrate needs to maximize glycogen stores.

If possible, meals should be times so they land 3–4 hours prior to a workout and should contain at least **60g of high-quality carbohydrate foods**, including whole-grains which will have time to digest and incorporate into muscle glycogen.

If you anticipate exercising in about an hour, consume **1–4 g/kg of high-glycemic, low fiber carbohydrates** which will be rapidly incorporated into liver and muscle glycogen. Examples include white bread, pasta, honey or a special sport gummy.

During exercise, you may consider consuming **30–60 g of carbohydrates** (*such as sport gels or gummies*) for exercise lasting longer than an hour, especially in intermittent (stop and go) sports like soccer, hockey and basketball.

After exercise, you should **replenish with 1.0 -1.2 g/kg of carbohydrates** (*alongside protein and fluids*) within 4–6 hours if you are exercising every day.

Protein

If you recall the chapter all about protein, you will remember that muscle-protein synthesis (MPS) is required for building muscle and increasing muscle mass. **MPS is stimulated by the ingestion of essential amino acids**, which are the building blocks of the protein we eat.

The key amino acid which plays a role in stimulating muscle-protein synthesis is the essential amino acid **leucine**. However, the effects of this amino acid work best when consumed as a complete protein, and not in isolation. This means that the whole foods you already eat, including animal and plant proteins are likely sufficient.

If your goals are muscle growth. protein supplementation has been shown to increase muscle growth and overall fat-free mass in resistance training programs lasting longer than 6-weeks.

If you decide to supplement, ensure your protein powder contains primarily **whey or pea protein isolates**. These isolates are complete sources of protein with the highest proportion of leucine.

What about Branched Chain Amino Acids (BCAAs?)

The branched-chain amino acids, leucine, isoleucine and valine are often packaged and sold as a nutritional supplement due to their MPS enhancing claims.

However, solely supplementing with BCAA's results in 50% less MPS compared to complete protein sources, as it is missing 5 out of the 9 essential amino acids. Remember that these the MPS properties of BCAA's work best when they are consumed in a complete protein.

How much protein should I eat before and after exercise?

Timing of protein consumption after exercise alongside adequate total daily protein intake is crucial for repairing muscles and stimulating muscle protein synthesis.

Within 1-hour after exercise, at least **20–30 g of protein,** containing **10 g of essential amino acids** should be consumed within 1-hour post exercise. Then, the timing of your next meal should be within 3–5 hours, as studies have shown that <u>MPS can only be maximally stimulated 3–5 hours apart.</u>

The recommended daily intake of protein for athletes is **1.2–2.0 g/kg/day** and MPS up-regulated for 24-hours following exercise. This means that consistent protein intake at all meal and snack opportunities is crucial for building muscle, especially for those who are exercising most days.

Fat and Ketogenic Diets

While we mostly think of glucose being the preferred source of fuel for our muscles, this starts to differ when we consider our aerobic metabolism and endurance athletes.

Athletes operating at lower intensity, or endurance exercise, will primarily oxidizing fat as their main source of energy. Endurance exercise includes swimming, distance running and biking.

Athletes at higher intensity are primarily oxidizing fat as their main source of energy, and function to reserve their glycogen stores for periodic bursts of energy if need be. This includes high-intensity interval training, weight-lifting, boxing and sprinting.

Following a low-carb, ketogenic diet for endurance athletes is known as *"training-low"*. Studies have shown that athletes who **<u>train low with a ketogenic diet *"up-regulate"* their fat oxidation enzymes</u>**, allowing to provide more energy from fat to fuel their muscles and enhance cellular outcomes of training.

You don't necessarily need to be following a low-carbohydrate ketogenic diet to achieve these effects, as the effects are not due to "ketosis" but rather the absence of available glycogen. For example, the same effects have been seen after performing <u>fasted cardio</u>, since glycogen stores are already low or depleted.

Why shouldn't resistance or strength training athletes follow a ketogenic diet?

When we "*up-regulate*" fat oxidation by following a ketogenic diet, we consequently "*down-regulate*" glucose oxidation, even when glycogen is available. This ultimately compromises the resistance or strength-training athletes as glucose most easily provides energy to our muscles under anaerobic stress.

However, remember that *not* choosing to follow a high-fat diet (such as a ketogenic diet) **does not mean that athletes should follow a low-fat diet**. Diets <20% energy from fat can risk deficiencies in essential omega-3 and omega-6 fatty acids.

Are sports nutrition supplements worth it?

Nutrition should always be optimized first through whole, high-quality foods. Whole foods are not comparable to supplements, and these products can never outweigh a bad diet, lack of sleep or poor training regimen.

However, some athletes may consider adding a nutritional supplement in their diet. If you live in the United States, remember that nutritional supplements are **not regulated**. Furthermore, supplements should always be consulted with your doctor and dietitian.

Creatine

What is it? Creatine is not a steroid. Creatine is an organic compound made from the amino acids glycine, arginine and methionine.

Our bodies create our own creatine, and creatine functions to provide our muscles with ATP (*the energy currency of our cells*). We also

consume creatine from animal protein, and studies have shown
that <u>vegetarians have lower levels of muscle creatine</u>.

What does it do? In high-intensity, anaerobic exercise our muscles
are depleted of ATP within 8–10 seconds. Creatine may help
prolong this period by supplying more ATP before it runs
out. <u>Studies</u> have supported creatine's positive effects on improving
muscles growth, performance enhancement and even cognitive
function.

How should I supplement? Creatine requires a loading period to
saturate muscles prior to taking effect. <u>The International Society of
Sports Nutrition</u> (ISSN) recommends 5 g of creatine 4x/day for 5–7
days, followed by maintenance at 3–5 g/day.

Absorption of the compound increases under the hormone insulin;
therefore it is recommended to consume with a protein/carb
containing meal. Creatine monophosphate is the most bioavailable
form of the supplement.

Antioxidant Supplements

What is it? Antioxidant supplements include omega-3 fatty acids
and vitamin C and E pills.

How does it work? Antioxidants are compounds naturally produced
by our body and can also be found in colourful fruits and vegetables.
They work by tackling oxidation by reducing *"reactive oxygen
species"* or ROS in our body. Antioxidant supplementation gained
momentum due to their claims on reducing inflammation and
speeding up recovery.

However, exercise is a natural inflammatory process, and athletes
adapt by increasing their own internal "antioxidant system". For
example, <u>trained athletes have higher levels of antioxidants
compared to untrained individuals</u>. But when we *"short-cut"* by

supplementing with antioxidants, we miss out on this adaptation.
This has been shown to worsen our bodies natural capabilities in
repairing muscles and recovery.

How should I supplement? Don't, and save your money. Focus on
eating foods after exercise high in antioxidants, including
blueberries, raspberries and dark leafy greens.

What happens when athletes don't consume enough energy? Introducing Relative Energy Deficit in Sports (RED-S)

RED-S is when athletes under-consume calories, compromises the
athlete's ability to perform in sport properly, and can have adverse
outcomes; diminished physiological functioning, decreased protein
synthesis and even adverse heart health.

Interestingly, consequences are more severe in female athletes
compared to male athletes. The International Olympic Committee
(IOC) has specifically outlined the nutritional consequences specific
to female athletes with RED-S, known as the "female-triad".

RED-S results in hormone dysregulation, resulting in irregular
menstrual functioning and poor bone health. These consequences are
detrimental to the growing female as the peak bone mineralization
period occurs during adolescence. This means that could stress
fractures that commonly occur in sports could be linked back to poor
nutrition. Therefore, when athletes encounter a stress fracture, they
may turn to physiotherapy, or ankle braces, but not treat the
underlying condition which is sub-optimal nutrition.

Furthermore, the increased energy expenditure which we exert on
our body when following a training regimen, combined with
insufficient caloric intake makes our body act a certain way. Our
body will begin to prioritize our energy for exercise, resulting for

decreased energy available for life processes, including protein synthesis, hormonal functioning and overall health.

Going back to female athletes, females are especially susceptible to eating disorders and issues with body image. Even if the body weight of active women is well within normal limits (and sometimes below), it is not uncommon for women to still want to maintain their below normal weight or lose that "extra" 5–10 lbs. Let's put this into a real-life example:

Julie is a 28-year-old female who exercises regularly. She is in great shape. She can easily run 10 km in 48 minutes or do an hour of intense training on the stair master, treadmill, or the elliptical machine. At 5'8", 140 lbs, her BMI is 20.7 and body fat 20%.

Julie is not overweight, yet she is unhappy with her weight and body shape. She meticulously watches what she eats and has hundreds of dieting tricks to take off that extra 5–7 lbs. Julie is successful at maintaining weight (but not losing). She skips meals, buys fat free snacks and diet sodas; she substitutes energy bars for meals; she avoids "bad" foods (any foods high in fat, calories, or sugar).

She has little variety in her diet. She frequently eats the same foods (types and amounts) daily. A special dinner out or an occasional dessert will bring on a bout of guilt—she will resume dieting or add an extra 1–2 miles into her daily run.

Sound familiar? With this cycle of restricting food intake with increased exercise, Julie is at a clear risk of developing RED-S.

To break this cycle, this woman, and other female athletes would actually benefit from an **increased caloric intake** to match energy expenditure. This is known as **reverse dieting**. Once Julie establishes sufficient food intake, she will be able to keep up to her body's energy demands, re-stabilize her hormones and promote muscle growth. Restabalization of hormones is crucial to maintain optimal bone mass and keep menstrual cycles regular. The importance of rest days should not be ignored, as these days are crucial for recovery and promoting muscle-protein synthesis to repair & grow new muscle tissue.

Sufficient caloric intake is also important for men. Within the context of bodybuilding or power performance sports, RED-S will also result in decreases testosterone and decrease muscle protein synthesis and overall poorer performance in sports and nutrition.

Many people may not achieve optimal energy intake for several reasons. It can be intentional, especially in weight-sensitive sports such as dance, volleyball and physique competition sports. It may also be due to poor planning, not consuming enough calories or even those who are food insecure or who are shopping on a tight food budget.

The bottom line: Adequate energy intake for athletes is imperative to avoid physiological consequences. Nutrition deficits may show-up later as injuries including bone fractures in athletes.

The Final Run-down

Sports nutrition can be complicated. However, remember that the cornerstone of proper nutrition is eating adequate calories, with quality carbohydrates, protein and fat. And don't undermine the power of proper sleep and hydration when it comes to maximizing performance.

The key nutritional takeaways you should remember from this chapter should include:

- Carbohydrates are crucial for high-intensity, anaerobic exercise including weight-lifting, HITT and sprinting. Consider eating 5–7 g/kg/day of carbohydrates.

- Protein intake is crucial throughout the entire day, and is higher for athletes. To optimize MPS, 20–30 g of protein should be consumed 2-hours after your workout.
- Low-carb, ketogenic diets may be beneficial for endurance athletes, as fat oxidation is their primary source of fuel.

Finally, remember that **sports nutrition is extremely individualized** for each athlete, as everyone's metabolism, gene expression, fitness level and medical history is different. Consultation with a sports dietitian is always the best source of information to improve your performance.

Chapter 3: Digestive Health

Digestive health has certainly been a buzzword over the last few years. With an increased number of gluten-free products available on the market and increased discussion around probiotics and prebiotics, could improving digestive health be the answer to all our health problems?

For those with a diagnosis of inflammatory bowel diseases, including crohn's and ulcerative colitis, intensive dietary management and close follow up with a team of medical professionals is imperative. Same with those diagnoses with celiac disease, an autoimmune disease that causes the gluten protein to trigger an immune response. But what triggers these diseases, and what about more minor digestive issues that everyone experiences?

In this chapter, we will go over the basics of digestive health, including the definitions of these diseases and the require intensive nutritional management and their health implications. We will also touch on other, common digestive health issues including non-celiac gluten sensitivity, bloating, gas, constipation and food sensitivities.

As digestive issues can be an indication of a more serious underlying health problems, always make sure that you consult with a health care professional prior making any major changes to your diet.

The digestive tract, or gastrointestinal tract, is a long, consistent tube that starts from our mouth and ends at our anus. The function of the digestive tract is to process, digest, absorb and excrete nutrients and energy. The digestive tract can be thought of the jetpack of our body, is it is the best way our body is able receive nutrition! The digestion system also includes other organs the help process nutrients, including the liver, gallbladder and the pancreas.

Fun Fact: *For hospitalized patients that are unable to eat for long periods of time, dietitians and doctors will begin a medical treatment known as enteral nutrition. Enteral nutrition is a tube that is threaded from the patients nose or mouth and ends in their stomach or small bowel. Artificial nutrition is infused into the digestive tract to keep them alive and to avoid weight-loss.*

When we consume food orally, our digestive system already gets to work by producing enzymes in our saliva to breakdown the sugars found in food. Once food is swallowed, it makes its way down the esophagus and into our stomach. Our stomach releases more enzymes and acidic juices to further breakdown the fats, proteins and sugars in our meal. The stomach acid is important to release certain nutrients, such as vitamin B12 to make sure they are more absorbable, or bio-available to our body.

Once our stomach has churned and broken down the food into absorbable parts, the food will reach our small intestine. The small intestine is full of small, finger-like projections known as villi and micro-villi. These villi are highly efficient at absorbing teeny-tiny nutrients and food components into the bloodstream.

Any indigestible food, such as fibres, will continue to the large intestine. Fibre can attract water, increasing the bulk and gel-like characteristics of our stool, helping us go to the bathroom. Fibre can also help reduce diarrhea, by absorbing extra water. Finally, stool is stored in the rectum that will be expelled during a bowel movement. Regular bowel movements are an important indicator of digestive health.

When something goes wrong in the digestive tract, some people may be diagnosed with digestive disease. For others, they may have a food sensitivity or have common symptoms after consuming certain foods. Let's go over some of the most serious, and less serious digestive issues and investigate how nutrition can help.

Ulcerative Colitis

Ulcerative colitis is a serious, autoimmune inflammatory bowel disease. The cause of ulcerative colitis is not completely understood and is often a combination of both genetic and environmental factors. For example, chronic stress and smoking has been linked to autoimmune diseases, including ulcerative colitis.

Fun Fact: *Autoimmune diseases mean that our body thinks that normal, body tissues and systems, such as the digestive tract are invaders. This causes our body to produce antigens against these body tissues, resulting in damage to the healthy tissue. There are many different reasons why an autoimmune disease may arise.*

Ulcerative colitis causes severe inflammation to the colon, or the large intestine. This can result in frequent diarrhea and may even present with blood or mucus in your stool. With this disease, it is hard for your body to properly absorb nutrients, and often results in weight-loss, nutrient deficiencies and malnutrition.

Crohn's Disease

Crohn's disease is very similar to ulcerative colitis, except it can occur anywhere in the digestive tract, from mouth to anus. Crohn's disease is slightly more common than ulcerative colitis and affects slightly more males than females. Similar to ulcerative colitis, both environmental and genetic factors can trigger the onset of the disease.

Crohn's disease triggers similar symptoms to ulcerative colitis, including diarrhea, blood in stool, a loss of appetite and nutrient deficiencies.

For both ulcerative colitis and crohn's disease, **it's important to note that food is not considered to cause the disease**, but once diagnosed , food can trigger flare-ups. Certain foods that are important to consume during **stable** periods of inflammatory bowel disease include protein-rich foods, fibrous foods and electrolyte drinks to help replenish electrolyte losses.

Celiac Disease & Gluten-Free Diets

Celiac disease has gained public awareness over the past few years mostly due to emerging, but conflicting research on the role of gluten in human health. For example, a Netflix documentary released in 2018 titled *"What's with Wheat"* spurred discussion as if everyone would benefit from removing gluten from their diet. These claims mostly arise from research conducted in rats, where the gluten protein, found in many grains, including wheat, rye and barley may contribute to a "leaky gut" resulting in systemic inflammation leading to a wide different range of health issues.

It's important to understand that humans are not rats, therefore it's important to weigh the risks and benefits of exclusion of such a staple ingredient, like bread, from our diet. Whole-grains provide a variety of nutrients important for human health, including fibre, B-vitamins and even beta-glucan, a type of fibre that is known for its power to lower cholesterol. Currently, there is not enough research to suggest that the benefits of not consuming whole grains outweigh the benefits of non-consuming wholegrains. In other words, for those who are not diagnosed with celiac disease or non-celiac gluten sensitivity, whole grains are perfectly fine for human health.

Celiac disease, on the other hand is a serious autoimmune disease to the protein gluten. Gluten proteins are primarily found in whole grains but can also be found in condiments, spices and even cosmetics. If a person with celiac disease consumes a food with gluten, their immune system will interpret it as an invader, and attack the protein which damages the intestinal tract.

For those living with celiac disease, a **gluten-free diet is one of the most effective ways to control and avoid symptoms.** Foods that do not include gluten include rice, amaranth, quinoa, buckwheat, corn, millet, sorghum and teff. Fruits and vegetables, meat, fish and dairy products area also gluten free. Following a strict gluten-free diet can be challenging, as there are many sources of gluten that are hidden. These hidden sources include canned foods, salad dressings and condiments, herbs and spices, vitamins and minerals and even candies. To note, beer contains gluten as it is fermented from wheat as well as soy sauce.

Oats, on the other hand are a topic of debate amongst nutrition scientists. Due to differing amounts of gluten due to cross-contamination, it is recommended that people living with celiac disease always purchase gluten free oats.

Non-Celiac Gluten Sensitivity

Unlike celiac disease, which requires a diagnosis based on the presence of antibodies to the protein gluten, some people present with gluten sensitivity in absence of antibodies to the gluten protein.

It is also different from diagnosed wheat-allergies, where serious allergic reactions can occur if an individual consumes wheat.

People with non-celiac gluten sensitivity often present with similar symptoms to those with celiac disease, including bloating, abdominal pain, acne and even weight-loss after consuming gluten-containing foods. This makes many individuals believe they may have celiac disease, when it is an intolerance to gluten.

The best way to manage non-celiac gluten sensitivity is through a food journal. If you believe you may have non-celiac gluten sensitivity, try eliminating all food sources of gluten in your diet for one week. In your food journal, which can be documented by pen and paper or through a mobile application, log your food entries and note your symptoms and how you feel during this week.

Even if you have non-celiac gluten sensitivity and your symptoms do not improve, it may take up to a month for symptoms to subside. If after two weeks, there are minimal improvements, try introducing 1-2 gluten containing foods into your diet to see if the symptoms worsen. If they do not worsen, keep consuming these foods and slowly introduce more foods until the symptoms improve or worsen. For certain individuals, different sources of gluten from different foods could be the triggering factor.

The Issue with Gluten-Free Diets

As mentioned above, there has been an explosion in the interest of gluten-free diets which has led to the development of many gluten-free products and brands on the market. While the removal of gluten from the diet has undeniable symptom improvement for those with non-celiac gluten sensitivity and a gluten-free diet is considered a medical treatment for celiac disease, **eliminating gluten from the diet of any individual could present with some downsides, including:**

Protein

Gluten is a protein, meaning when it is removed from whole grains, the protein content of the whole grain is decreased. For example, one slice of normal gluten-containing bread provides about 4-6 grams of protein. This means that in a sandwich with two slices of bread will contain an additional 8-12 grams of protein, while gluten-free bread typically provides 0-2 grams of protein per slice.

Fortification and B-Vitamins

In certain countries, like Canada, it is mandatory for flour, which is the main ingredient in gluten-containing breads, to be fortified with B-vitamins, including folate. Folate is especially in important vitamin for pregnant women and soon-to-be pregnant women. This B-vitamin is crucial for the embryonic development and to prevent neural tube defects. Without proper levels of folate, the neural tube of fetuses can become underdeveloped, leading to severe birth defects.

Expensive Diet

When purchasing gluten-free breads, flours and specialty items, the diet can be significantly more expensive than gluten-containing products. This means for those on a limited budget, eating a gluten-free diet can be heavy on the wallet. In fact, an analysis study revealed that on average, gluten-free products are 242% more expensive than regular, gluten-containing products. For those who absolutely do not need to exclude gluten, keeping gluten in your diet can make more financial sense.

Other Food Sensitivities

On the other hand, some people experience intolerances to foods that may be attributed to irritable bowel syndrome, or IBS. Unlike crohn's, ulcerative colitis and celiac disease, irritable bowel syndrome is not a diagnosed disease or disorder but rather an umbrella of common digestive symptoms that many people experience.

The symptoms of IBS are very general, and include frequent gas, stomach cramps, bloating, constipation and diarrhea. For mild cases of IBS, it may be worthwhile to follow a low FODMAP (pronounced FAWD-MAP) diet.

This diet targets common fermentable sugars found in the diet that can trigger digestive problems. These undigested carbohydrates are fermented in the large intestine, which can produce gas and cause cramping. They can also have an osmotic pull, meaning they pull water into the digestive tract and cause diarrhea.

A low FODMAP diet helps eliminate the most common food triggers for IBS, helping individuals reduce their symptoms while still enjoying a wide variety of foods. If you suffer from minor IBS symptoms, including gas, stomach cramps and bloating you can **try a low FODMAP diet for 4-8 weeks**, and then slowly re-introduce the different types of fermentable sugars into your diet to pin-point which ones you are sensitive to.

What is the low FODMAP diet?

FODMAP is an acronym that stands for the most common fermentable sugars that can trigger food sensitivities. These include:

1) **Oligosaccharides:** These sugars include those found in wheat, rye, legumes, garlic and onions. Wheat and rye are most often found in breads, baked goods and cereals. Legumes include chickpeas, lentils, black beans, kidney

beans, pinto beans, peas and peanuts (including peanut
butter!).

> **Suggested Swaps:** Onions are the flavour basis of
> many important dishes. Some suggested swaps
> include the green tips of green-onions and chives,
> leeks and fennel. You can also try using the Indian
> spice asafoetida which has a pungent taste similar to
> onions. For garlic, you can try using garlic oil. For
> legumes, which are an important source of plant-
> based protein can be replaced with tofu. You can also
> consume small amounts of legumes, like chickpeas
> and lentils by rinsing the legumes well. This process
> helps remove some of the oligosaccharide content.
> For grains, you can consume millet, quinoa, brown
> rice, oats and tapioca.

2) **Disaccharides:** These sugars include those found in milk,
   yogurt and soft cheeses, mainly from the sugar lactose, which
   most of the population cannot digest as our bodies reduce or
   shut-off the production of the enzyme lactase shortly after
   stopping breastfeeding. The reason that more Americans are
   able to digest lactose is due to a genetic adaption brought
   over by European settlers, however lactose intolerance is
   more prevalent across other cultures, including Asian and
   Middle Eastern.

> **Suggested Swaps:** To avoid lactose, you can
> purchase lactose-free milks. You can also try dairy-
> free milks including almond milk and cashew milk.
> Other dairy-free milks including soy milk and oat
> milk are higher in FODMAPS but can be consumed
> in small amounts.

3) **Monosaccharides:** These sugars include figs, mangoes and
   natural sweeteners such as honey and agave. In these foods,
   fructose is the main fermentable sugar in these foods. All
   fruits contain fructose, but in differing amounts.

> **Suggested Swaps:** Natural maple syrup (not the Aunt Jemimah's kind) has a lower ratio of fructose content, meaning it is a more suitable and natural sweetened swap for higher FODMAP sweeteners. Low-FODMAP fruits include blueberries, kiwi, citrus fruits, pineapple and strawberries.

4) And **Polyols:** Polyols are sugar alcohols, including mannitol and sorbitol that is found in certain foods including blackberries and low-calorie sweeteners, including sugar-free gum. Polyols can also be found in some vegetables including asparagus, brussel sprouts, cauliflower, mushrooms and artichokes.

> **Suggested Swaps:** Avoid chewing sugar-free gum, swap out blackberries with blueberries and try low-FODMAP vegetables, including bean sprouts, red pepper, kale, tomato, spinach and zucchini.

If you haven't caught on already, following the low FODMAP diet can be tricky as there are many rules and exceptions. Additionally, eliminating foods found on the low FODMAP diet can actually have negative health consequences as most foods containing FODMAPS are generally healthy foods. These fruits, vegetables, plant-proteins and whole grains are an important source of antioxidants, vitamins & minerals, protein, fibre and prebiotics that are integral to supporting good health.

It's important to note that most people are not sensitive to all FODMAPS, and only specific foods that are high in FODMAPS, and following a restrictive diet that eliminates all these food sources is not sustainable or healthy. This is why if you decide to start a low FODMAP diet, be sure to consult a professional such as a Registered Dietitian to customize the plan for your needs.

The (not-so-much) Science Behind Food Sensitivity Tests

Perhaps you have been scrolling through social media and an ad pops up that suggests by sampling your blood, breath or urine they will be able to diagnose all your food sensitivities. These companies, inspired by the real challenge's individuals face in combating their digestive problems can be misleading when it comes to a real solution to solve these issues. The truth is that these food sensitivity tests are based <u>in extremely limited science</u> and are overhyped on emerging evidence and may cause problems where people believe they need to restrict many foods to overcome their symptoms.

One of the most commonly available commercial food sensitivity tests is an Immunoglobulin G (IgG) food test. In these tests, a sample of your blood will be analyzed for IgG, which is a type of antibody. However, scientific evidence does not support the use of this test to identify individual foods as the **antibody IgG is produces as a normal response to food ingestion**. In fact, <u>science suggests</u> that higher levels of IgG after ingestion of food indicates that your body is processing food **properly** and not improperly.

There are also concerns with the test is confusing people between allergies and insensitivities. For example, if someone is allergic to a certain food, their levels of IgG for this food may be lower. If this person were to take an unregulated food sensitivity test, their IgG levels for their allergen may be reported as low and they would be told they are not sensitive to this food, while in reality they could have a life-threatening allergy.

Furthermore, the pricing of some of these tests can range between $400-$700, quite a pretty penny for a test that is based in virtually no scientific evidence with limited reports of improved patient symptoms after removing their foods from their diet.

Our verdict? Skip the food sensitivity tests and speak with a Registered Dietitian who may suggest you try a low FODMAP diet instead of a pricey food sensitivity test. It's also important to take care of your gut microbiome to be proactive in limiting the development of these digestive issues, which will be covered in the next chapter.

Chapter 4: The Gut Microbiome

Who would have thought that 2020 would be the year where a teeny, tiny, invisible microorganism would take the world by storm? While a certain virus is threatening health infrastructure and populations at a global level, other invisible colonies are working hard to keep our environment, health and wellbeing in balance.

Microorganisms exist in a world where there is power in their numbers. For example, microorganisms existing in our own body outweigh our own human cells 10:1, over 100 trillion bacteria reside solely in our gut and make up an estimated 1–3% of our total body mass.

Microbes have also existed for billions of years, colonizing our planet long before the human race. Therefore, the ecosystem we are evolving to have with these teeny tiny organisms is—relatively speaking—only recently becoming uncovered.

What is our microbiome?

Different communities of microbes populate different areas of our body, not just in our gut. For example, a certain bacterium found on our skin produces toxins to combat harmful bacteria. On the other hand, colonization of the skin with the bacterium *C. acnes* results in problematic pimples and gives rise to the feared teenaged aesthetic— acne.

Bacteria inhabiting our mouth will secrete substances to lower pH, which creates an acidic environment to help ward off other cavity-causing bacterial species. The microbiota of both male and female reproductive tracts helps create a defence against sexually-transmitted infections, yeast infections and urinary-tract infections.

And you're correct in thinking that the reproductive microbiota of one partner can influence that of the other.

Our gut is thought to house over 100 trillion microbes, home to the most diversity and abundance out of all other body parts. Our gut microbiome plays a crucial role in <u>nutrient metabolism and immune defence,</u> and is referred to as a "*microbial organ*" due these complex and important functions.

Collectively, these different communities of microbes inhabiting different parts of our bodies create our own **microbiome.** While we share about 99.9% of our genome with the rest of humankind on earth, our <u>microbiomes can be up to 80–90% different.</u>

Therefore, you can think of your microbiome as your own **personalized microbial fingerprint**, different from any other human being in the world.

What influences our microbiome?

Our first inoculation with microbes starts at birth through the vaginal canal and continues with breastfeeding. For life beyond infancy, our microbiome blueprint highly depends on our individual lifestyle and environment. This includes our geographical region, who we live with, our age, medical history, age and diet—just to name a few.

Scientists have coined the term "*dysbiosis*" to refer to when our microbiome is disrupted or off balance. These disruptions may contribute to the development of metabolic and auto-immune diseases, including obesity, inflammatory bowel disease and even cancer.

Various environmental triggers, including changes in diet and lifestyle patterns or encountering health problems, such as infections which require courses of antibiotics can disrupt the complex microbial make-up of our microbiome.

However, everyone's microbiome is extremely complex and different, and scientists and clinicians do not yet have an exact definition as to what a healthy or normal microbiome is. This means that there is no robust evidence for clinicians to start diagnosing or treating people with microbiomes out of balance.

Can I change my gut microbiome through diet?

When we rewind our anthropological clock, researchers highlight how ancestral humans ate a diet rich in plants and plant roots, which inherently includes a lot of indigestible fibres. These indigestible fibres are known as **prebiotics** and promote the growth of beneficial bacterial strains such as lactobacillus and bifidobacteria. These microbes and foods work together to help promote and maintain a healthy gut microbiome.

Research has also demonstrated that our gut microbiome responds rapidly to changes in diet composition, especially when switching between animal and plant-based diets. Evolutionarily speaking, this makes sense as we used to intermittently feast on animal protein, then fall back on plant foods in times of caloric and nutrient scarcity.

Strong research has demonstrated that our gut microbiome responds rapidly to changes in diet composition, especially when switching between animal and plant-based diets.

Our diets are now heavily influenced by industrialization, and for those privileged to choose what to eat each day, we can devour a wide-range of food groups coming from both animal and plant-based sources and even probiotics. Ultimately, different diets are seen to alter the ratio of the two-dominating phylum in our gut microbiome—*Bacteroidetes and Firmicutes.*

Plant-based Diets and the Gut Microbiome

Plant-based diets are rich in vegetables, fruits, whole grains, nuts and seeds. Most plant foods contain fibre, where these indigestible carbohydrates are fermented into beneficial short-chain fatty acids. Polyphenols found in plants may also increase bifidobacteria and lactobacillus bacterium which are thought to have anti-inflammatory effects.

Research has drawn associations between plant-based diets and increased microbial diversity, especially with an increased amount of *Bacteroidetes* compared to *Firmicutes*. This diversity and increased ratio have been associated with maintaining a health body weight.

People living with obesity and with higher BMIs have been shown to have *less* diversity and a *higher* amount of Firmicutes. However, evidence is limited, and opposite results have also been found.

Animal-based Diets and the Gut Microbiome

Diets based heavily around animal protein have seen to have the opposite effects of plant-based diets. They decrease overall microbial diversity and have been seen to increase the amount of *Firmicutes*. The Firmicutes phylum may extract up to an additional 150 calories of energy from the digestion process which can lead to weight-gain overtime.

One study where participants consumed a diet of eggs, bacon, beef, pork and cheese ad libitum for 5 days found an increase in bile-tolerant microorganisms. This may be partly due to the fact that bile acids are produced proportionally to the amount of fat we eat.

Studies conducted on animals have hypothesized that an increase in bile acids caused by a high-fat animal diet could negatively impact our gut microbiome. Secondary by-products of bile acids are pro-inflammatory and have been linked to the development of inflammatory bowel disease. However, similar to the studies with plant-based diets, these results are inconsistent.

Does this mean plant-based diets are good, and animal-based diets are bad?

It is important to note that we are very early on in understanding the gut microbiome and its response to changing our diet. As previously mentioned, contradicting results have been found in both plant-based and animal-based diets with respect to the gut microbiome.

Much of what we know about the gut microbiome stems from lower-quality evidence, such as those in mice models and associative epidemiological studies.

Therefore, while these preliminary findings can seem like they hold all the answers to resolve obesity or inflammatory bowel disease—they only paint part of the picture. Remember that the microorganisms which co-exist in our body are enormous in number and highly complex. They are influenced by *many* different factors—**diet is just one of them.**

Ultimately, future high-quality studies are required so scientists can further their understanding of what a healthy gut microbiome really is, and how to treat those that are not. Until then—you are likely fine eating a healthy balanced diet rich in vegetables, fruits, whole grains, nuts, seeds and protein foods.

Next, lets dive into the world of probiotics.

What are the scientifically proven health benefits of probiotics & prebiotics?

Probiotics are the live microorganisms that exits in our digestive tract, primarily in the colon. Prebiotics are the "food" for these microorganisms. We consume prebiotics almost every day, through the consumption of indigestible fibres. Both probiotics and prebiotics play an important role in establishing a healthy gut microbiome.

It's difficult to tease out all the different effects of probiotics, as there are many different strains of bacteria and yeasts which cause different health effects. A lot of studies on probiotics have been 'in-vitro" (or done in a laboratory or test-tube) and are not necessarily scalable to humans.

Furthermore, everyone's gut microbiome is different, and scientists have not yet defined what a "*normal*" or "*optimal*" gut microbiome, therefore we haven't established a baseline to yet treat certain diseases or health problems.

However, although it's difficult to prescribe or recommend any specific strain to prevent or treat a certain issue. Consuming a healthy diet which contains different sources of probiotics and prebiotics can still have real health benefits, including:

Effects on the Gut Microbiome

As previously discussed, the gut microbiome plays numerous roles in human health, including energy balance and immune response. Disruption of our normal gut microbiome can result in something known as dysbiosis which is associated with numerous metabolic diseases, including obesity, inflammatory bowel diseases and cancer.

Consuming prebiotics and probiotics can promote the growth of good bacteria in our gut microbiome, leading to better digestion and improved overall health.

Effects on Weight-Loss

People with dysbiosis may have a greater disadvantage of losing weight, especially if they are already obese as their gut microbiome is found to be less diverse. For example, they might possess certain type of microbes which extract more calories during digestion than those of a normal weight. In one study, people with dysbiosis and obesity extracted an extra 400 calories per day.

Consuming prebiotics and probiotics can help decrease this dysbiosis, and potentially aid in weight-loss.

Effects on Immunity

Our gut is responsible for a large part of our innate immune system. Our gut protects us from outside bad bacteria by having a rich mucus lined surface and a relatively impermeable intestinal barrier.

Probiotics can attach to the mucosal surface of our gut to increase the amount of mucous and even create a slightly more acidic environment which lessens the chances of harmful bacteria and pathogens surviving. It can also prevent the binding of harmful pathogens in our gut and preventing what is known as "leaky gut". Prebiotics will ensure the survival of these beneficial probiotics.

However, just because these foods can have impacts on the immune system in our gut the cellular level, it does not translate into boosting immunity against other infectious diseases, such as COVID-19 which is a respiratory illness which attacks other receptors in our lungs.

Ultimately, consuming a source of probiotics and prebiotics do have beneficial effects on health, but require an overall healthy and active lifestyle to reap the reward. That being said, try including the following sources of pre and probiotics in your diet regularly:

Prebiotics

- Apples

- Underripe Bananas

- Asparagus

- Mushrooms

- Oats

- Garlic and Onions

Probiotics

- Yogurt made with probiotic strains including Bifidobacterium and lactobacillus

- Kefir

- Sauerkraut

- Kimchi

- Miso

- Sourdough bread

Chapter 5: Mental Health & Nutrition

Introduction to Mental Health & Nutrition

Mental health is a serious health issue for many individuals. Throughout 2020 and continuing into 2021, the signature of the global pandemic was not only the lockdowns, social isolation, job losses and health insecurity – but also brought on an unprecedented mental health crisis. Whether one was already living with a mental illness or the stress of the pandemic triggered the onset of a brand new one, it is undeniable that the global health crisis has a tremendous impact on our day to day lives.

You may be wondering, what is the link between all this and nutrition? The truth is that nutrition and mental health have a bi-directional relationship. In other words, what we eat can impact our mental state and our mental state can impact what we eat.

Let's stay on topic regarding the coronavirus pandemic. In July of 2020, a national survey conducted in the United States revealed that 53% of adults mental health was negatively impacted due to the pandemic. As a result, their overall wellbeing and motivation also decreased, with 32% struggling to eat regularly and 12% with increased alcohol consumption or substance use. Here we can see a direct correlation between poor mental health and lifestyle habits. Why so? Let's turn to the science to discuss.

The link between mental health impacting nutrition

Keeping individuals mentally healthy and happy is a huge public health priority. In fact, it is estimated that mental illnesses carry one of the world's highest burden of disease, outpacing other diseases including cardiovascular disease and cancer. Depression, a mental illness characterized by the loss of interest in day-to-day activities and excessive fatigue is a predictor of lower diet quality, meaning that those with less energy throughout the day are less likely to be able to cook healthy meals. In fact, a high-quality cross sectional study supports this association.

This means that when poor mental health arrives first to the scene, good nutrition and healthy habits are one of the first things to go, which can further depreciate mood. Some people may be inclined to overeat, while others many are not able to eat at all. A few of these mental changes may be explained by physical changes going on in the brain during periods of stress, depression or anxiety.

Our appetite is largely regulated by the hypothalamus, a part of our brain that triggers the release of both hunger and fullness hormones.

<u>Some studies</u> suggest that during periods of stress, fullness hormones are less efficient in letting our brains know we have eaten enough and can trigger overeating.

Furthermore, psychological stress elicits the release of the stress hormone cortisol. Cortisol stimulates the release of glucose, or sugar, into the bloodstream. From an evolutionary standpoint this response makes sense: If we were face to face with a predator (stress), we would need energy (sugar) to fight the predator or run away. This is known as the **fight-or-flight response** that has allowed us to outrun and fight off dangerous predators. Today, this fight-or-flight response may be triggered by psychological stress such as reading the news or losing a lost one. In this state of chronic stress, high levels of cortisol in our blood may also trigger overeating.

On the other hand, activation of the stress response can also cause the opposite effect: undereating or a total loss of appetite. While science is not completely sure why some people overweight and others undereat during stressful periods, undereating could be partly explained by the activation of the **sympathetic nervous system**.

As introduced above, our fight or flight response is a response to stress. This response triggers the activation of the sympathetic nervous system, which essentially tells our body to constrict our blood vessels to our heart, lungs and brain and decrease blood flow to other organs, including our digestive, reproductive and urinary systems. This is why when we are stressed, our heart beats faster, our breathing increases and some may even be able to think quicker. However, decreased blood flow to our digestive system means that we may have difficulties sensing hunger signals and digesting and enjoying food. As a result, food intake can decrease, and undereating occurs.

Ultimately, a cyclical pattern begins to emerge where depressed, stressed or anxious moods results in unhealthy eating patterns which reinforces the altered mental state.

How to break this cycle? Be sure to speak with a registered psychologist or a doctor for professional mental health advice. On the other hand, here are a few suggestions that may help encourage healthful food choices during stressful, anxious and uncertain times:

Identify high energy and low energy days

While relative to each individual, we all have our higher and lower energy days, or even hours throughout the day. When a whiff of motivation or energy is in the air, try taking this time to prepare a healthy meal or meal prep for the week ahead.

Some people may experience slightly higher energy in the mornings, while others may be more energetic on Fridays. Whatever it is, try paying attention to your body and your mood carefully to identify even an hour of slightly higher energy.

For easy and healthy recipe ideas, try out some of these:

- **English Muffin Pizzas:** Preheat the oven the 350 F. On a baking sheet, spread 2 tablespoons of pizza sauce on an open-faced english muffin. Add a few vegetables, including tomato, red pepper, onion or mushrooms and then cover with ¼ cup of shredded cheese. Bake for 10-15 minutes and enjoy mini pizzas!

- **Chicken Burrito Bowls:** Preheat the oven to 375 F. On a baking sheet lined with tin foil, place 2-4 chicken breasts and season with store-bought taco seasoning (or make your own with salt, pepper, cumin, paprika and chili powder) and lime juice. Bake for 25-30 minutes or until the internal temperature reaches at least 165 F. Then, add chicken to a bowl of rice and top with beans, guacamole, salsa, cheese and sour cream.

- **Protein Smoothies:** Add 1 scoop of protein powder, a handful of nuts, 2 tablespoons of chia seeds, ½ cup of Greek Yogourt or 2 tablespoons of nut butter to any smoothie to increase its protein content. This protein will power you with the energy you need for the day while giving you a punch of antioxidants from any fruit you add.

- **Pre-Cut Fruit & Veggies:** While this one may not be the most exciting, making healthy foods accessible and easing to consume is one of the best ways to improve eating habits! After you purchase your groceries each week, try cutting carrots, cucumber, celery and red pepper into bite size slices and store in the refrigerator. Same goes for pre-washing berries, slicing watermelon or even freezing bananas to easily add them into smoothies.

Practice mindful and intentional eating

Have you ever sat in front of the TV with a snack, such as a bowl of ice cream or a bag of chips and all of a sudden, you realized you ate the entire thing without even getting a chance to enjoy it? Since you didn't get to enjoy it you wander back to the cupboard to replace the snack you just ate, and the process repeats itself. This is known as mind*less* or *unintentional* eating, where instead of sitting down and appreciate the food we are eating, we do quite the opposite.

Mindful and intentional eating requires that one is focused entirely on the experience of the meal, including before, after and during the eating event. Some tips to bring awareness to mealtimes include asking yourself the following questions:

1) **Why?** Ask yourself "why am I eating?". Are you able to physiologically feel signs of hunger? Are you tired, stressed or bored? Why did you choose this specific food or meal? Is it special to you or important?

This first question triggers the limbic system, a part of your brain that is responsible for emotions and feelings. By asking yourself "why?" you can get to the root cause as to why you have decided to eat in this very moment. Of note, there is not perfect answer to "why" you are eating but asking "why" brings an important awareness to the eating event.

2) **What?** Ask yourself "what am I eating?". Is this your favourite food? What individual ingredients went into the making of this meal? What are your feelings about this food you are about to eat?

Truly identifying what you are eating can help you connect with the food in front of you. By bringing awareness to each individual ingredient, you can establish appreciation for the foods you are about to eat.

3) **Where?** Ask yourself "where will I be eating this?". Will it be snuggled up on your couch watching your favourite movie, or will it be at the dinner table next to your family?

Similar to the above, there is no right or wrong answer to where one should be eating. For some, eating in front of the TV will bring joy after a long week while eating together as a family will foster connection. The key is bringing awareness and intention to where you are eating.

4) **How?** Ask yourself "how will I be eating this?". Is it with a fork or a spoon, or will it just be with your hands? Does it need to be cut up into little bits? Will it be messy, or relatively simple?

While it might seem silly, identifying how you will eat the meal also establishes awareness of the eating experience. Answering this small question can lead to big appreciations of the little things, including having the dexterity to eat a sandwich, or the money to purchase stainless steel forks and soft napkins.

Eat together

Although it was previously mentioned that there is no best *place* to eat a meal, it may be better to eat with others rather than alone. Throughout evolution, eating and sharing food has always been a social experience. Eating different foods can even express personality traits and cultural preferences.

Experts recommend that eating together can result in less overeating and even improve overall mood. While we hope that restrictions on social gatherings may ease throughout 2021, a simple phone call over a meal or even sending a photo of your meal over text can instill social connection.

Find inspiration

Sometimes, all we need is a bit of inspiration to spark our motivation to try out a new yummy recipe or try meal prepping for the first time. Try searching YouTube, Pinterest and even Tik Tok for meal inspiration. Just be wary of those giving out nutrition advice if they are not qualified nutritionists or dietitians.

Hydrate

In the end, make sure that you are well hydrated throughout the day. Not drinking enough water can cause fatigue and headaches. Try carrying a water bottle with you at all times to remind yourself to drink water. On average, most people need at least 25-30 ml per kilogram of body weight.

Now that we've uncovered why eating habits are impacted by changes in mood, and different strategies to combat these changes, it's equally important to discuss the other direction that exists in the relationship between nutrition and mental health: specific foods and nutrients that could directly have **an impact on brain function and mental health.**

Fruits & Vegetables

A systematic review analyzed the associations between fruit and vegetable intake and mental health in adults and revealed that certain subgroups of fruits and vegetables, including **berries, citrus, and green leafy vegetables** could promote higher levels of optimism and self-efficacy. In fact, one study that controlled for other lifestyle factors, including exercise and smoking, found that a higher intake of fruits and vegetables had the strongest association with better mental health.

It is recommended that adults should have at least 8-10 portions of fruits and vegetables per day, and these levels are considered to play a role in preserving or improving mental health. Scientists still aren't entirely sure why certain foods, or nutrients can influence mental health. But they do have a couple guesses as to why these everyday foods can have a powerful impact. Let's dig in.

Antioxidants

Berries, citrus fruits and red, orange and green leafy vegetables are high in something known as **antioxidants.** Antioxidants include a wide range of vitamins, including vitamin C, E and A, and are thought to play a role in helping to reduce **brain inflammation**.

Inflammation is a normal body process. It occurs when we eat, when we exercise and even when we sleep. If we emerge ourselves into the human body, normal chemicals can transform themselves into a free radical, which is an altered form of oxygen known as a superoxide.

These superoxides travel around the body producing inflammation as they damage cells. Our body has our own antioxidant, or superoxide-fighting system, that disarms this molecule and neutralizes the inflammation.

Lack of sleep, stress and poor nutrition can decrease the effectiveness of this antioxidant system and high inflammation is associated with mental illnesses. This means that consuming foods high in antioxidants may help supplement our body's own antioxidant system, fighting off inflammation and potentially improving overall mental health.

The bottom line? Eat your vegetables and fruits, especially berries, leafy green vegetables like kale and spinach and orange/red vegetables, like red peppers and carrots.

Pre and Probiotics

As mentioned in the chapter all about digestive health, pre and probiotics play a powerful role in our gut microbiome. As a quick refresher, prebiotics are indigestible fibres that serve as food for the beneficial bacteria in our gut. Examples of prebiotics include oats, apples, asparagus, mushrooms, garlic and onions. Probiotics are beneficial, live microorganisms. Examples of foods that contain probiotics include yogurts, kefir, sauerkraut and kimchi.

Through the gut brain axis, beneficial compounds produced by the bacteria in our gut can help preserve the intestinal barrier, decreasing inflammation throughout the body. This decreased inflammation may decrease the stress hormone, cortisol.

Furthermore, our gut microbiota helps in the synthesis of serotonin, the happy hormone synthesized from tryptophan found in our diet.

Let's talk more about the production of serotonin and the link with nutrition.

Tryptophan and B vitamins

Our gut-brain axis is influenced by the activity in our gut and in our brain. One component of our mood is influenced by the amount of serotonin produced in our brain. Those with lower levels of serotonin often experience depressed mood, lack of motivation, trouble focusing and fatigue. However, in order to create serotonin, our brain first needs **tryptophan.**

Tryptophan is an amino acid, or a building block of the proteins we consume in our diet. Tryptophan is found in nearly all foods but can be found in slightly higher amounts in animal meats, plant proteins and nuts & seeds.

When tryptophan is released from protein foods through digestion, it will become converted to serotonin by our gut microbiota with the help of two important B-vitamins: **Folate and Vitamin B12**.

Folate is commonly found in fortified in whole grain breads and cereals, while vitamin B12 is almost exclusively found in animal-based foods or speciality fortified plant-based foods, such as fortified plant milk or nutritional yeast. If you are following a vegetarian or vegan diet, it is important to take a vitamin B12 supplement to make sure you are able to produce enough serotonin.

Once tryptophan is converted into serotonin with the help of its two B vitamins: Folate & vitamin B12, it will cross the blood-brain barrier and will travel to the brain to play its role in regulating mood, fatigue, cognition and in studies where levels of tryptophan are depleted in humans, serotonin production halts to a stop and results in lower mood.

The bottom line? Make sure you are eating enough protein, plant-based or animal based and consume whole grains. If you follow a plant-based diet, make sure you are consuming enough vitamin B12 or take a daily supplement.

Zinc, Magnesium and Selenium

Some studies have made links between lower levels of zinc, magnesium and selenium with higher levels of depression in a population.

Zinc is a mineral found in foods such as red meat, seafood, legumes, nuts and dairy products. Zinc helps assist the millions of chemical reactions and processed in the brain that are responsible for neuron growth and brain function.

Researchers suspect that zinc can regulate the synapsis of neurotransmitters in the brain, decreasing the release of the stress hormone cortisol and act as an antioxidant to decrease inflammation.

 In a systematic review of randomized-control trials, human participants who consumed a zinc supplement daily reported experiencing an overall improved mood with less depressive symptoms. However, some of these studies combined zinc and anti-depressants, and did not evaluate zinc alone so it's hard to tell if mood truly improved with the addition of the zinc supplement.

Magnesium is a micronutrient found in green leafy vegetables, nuts, seeds and whole grains. Magnesium is crucial for helping processes in our central nervous system, including our brain. It is suggested that magnesium can activate a receptor in the brain that is associated with memory and cognition, but changes in mood have only been reported in rat studies.

Selenium is an essential trace element that is essential for the production of powerful antioxidants in our brain and nervous system.

Whole grains, nuts and seeds are a good source of selenium, especially brazil nuts. The role that selenium plays in mental health has many theories, but one is linked to our thyroid.

Our thyroid gland is a small, butterfly shaped organ located in the middle of our neck. It is responsible for producing the active thyroid hormone, T3, which regulates many metabolic processes of the body.

Selenium helps to synthesize the T3 hormone, and lower levels of T3 cause hypothyroidism, which is linked to weight-gain, fatigue and depression. Of note, iodine, found in iodized salt, fish, dairy products and seaweed is also a crucial mineral required for T3 synthesis.

Bottom Line: Enjoy 1-2 brazil nuts per day for selenium and ensure you are consuming a source of iodine each day, such as from fish, dairy products or seaweed.

L-Theanine

While it may sound fancy, L-theanine is simply a type of amino acid found in green tea. It is most well-known for its calming and anti-anxiety effects, but is this supported by science?

A 2020 systematic review of the effects of L-theanine found that a supplementation of 200-400 mg/day of the amino acid reduced stress and anxiety compared to placebo in individuals already pre-exposed to stress. However, these were in relatively small studies, and other trials show different results.

Bottom Line: L-theanine is found in green tea, a drink that has been consumed for thousands of years and known for its powerful antioxidant properties. In addition, it provides a burst of caffeine that can stimulate mood and energy. Whether L-theanine works or not, green tea definitely has health benefits that make it worth drinking a few cups per day.

Vitamin D

Vitamin D made headlines in 2020 and will likely continue to do so in 2021. Throughout the coronavirus pandemic, 33-97% of severely ill patients infected with COVID-10 admitted to the Intensive Care Unit (ICU) had vitamin D deficiency. The mortality rate of those deficient in vitamin D was also much higher, where one study found a 21% mortality rate for Vitamin D deficient COVID-19 patients compared to 3.1% with normal vitamin D levels.

So, what is vitamin D? Known as the "sunshine vitamin", Vitamin D can be synthesized through our skin, turning inactive compounds into a powerful vitamin that is essential for many body functions. However, those with darker skin or who are living in colder climates with less yearly sunshine are at higher risk of vitamin D deficiency. Vitamin D is also found sparingly in food, with small amounts found in eggs, fortified milk and meat products and margarine.

Vitamin D is not just a vitamin, but also acts as a hormone known as *cholecalciferol*. This hormone can enter into our cells and turn on an off gene that can influence how we interact and respond to our environment. It can also regulate calcium absorption into our bones, preserving bone health.

While widely considered to play a universal role in mood, a 2020 systematic review of randomized controlled trials found that vitamin D supplementation may only improve depressive symptoms in those diagnosed with clinical depression and not in others without a diagnosis. In a 2020 randomized control trial with over 18,000 adults, vitamin D supplementation did not improve depressive symptoms in the general population.

Bottom Line: Vitamin D is tremendously important to human health, and many people are deficient in the vitamin due to lack of sunlight, lack of foods naturally high in vitamin D and darker skin colours. While there may not be a direct link between vitamin D levels and mental health, its recommended to consume a daily supplement to meet your needs.

In terms of mental health, is food medicine?

While this chapter went extensively over the different vitamins, minerals and trace minerals that have been found to impact our brain and influence mental health, there is an important message to get across: Nutrition, food and a healthy diet may play one of many roles in maintaining good mental health. Food is not medicine, but food and proper nutrition can be one strategy when it comes to mental health.

Maintaining good mental health is mutli-factorial, and depends on genetics, environment and other lifestyle factors, including getting regular exercise, not smoking and managing stress. **Mental illnesses are serious, and stem much deeper than individual diet**. However, the good news remans that there is emerging evidence that foods can have an effect on our mental state, and food can be a coping strategy when it comes to managing stress, anxiety and depression.

If you are struggling with a mental illness, make sure you speak to a psychologist and your family doctor about incorporating a few of the strategies discussed in this chapter.

Chapter 6: Trendy Dietary Patterns in 2021 – Myths & Facts

2020 was a world where misinformation took the world by storm. Continuing into 2021, the media and influencers swirl different diets over the news and social media platforms nearly every single day, leading to a lot of confusion about what the best type of diet there is to consume.

In this chapter, we will go over some of the common myths and facts that surround these diets, including low carbohydrate and vegan and vegetarian diets. With this information in hand, this chapter should arm you with the knowledge to decide what diet is best for you to follow, or not to follow.

Trendy Dietary Pattern #1 : Low Carbohydrate Diets

If you're even somewhat well versed in today's *"nutritional pop-culture"* you have likely seen that carbohydrates, whole-grains, cereals, starchy vegetables, fruit and sweetsor anything composed of glucose, is very much out of style.

This also conveniently coincides with the rising incidence of people living with obesity, hypertension, type II diabetes or other cluster of metabolic risks which are known as *metabolic syndrome.*

 Many self-proclaimed "nutrition coaches", doctors with minimal nutritional education or individuals with promising success stories currently dominate the nutritional main-stream media, offering a glimmer of hope in an era of metabolic despair—***could the low-carbohydrate diet be the answer to all of our nutritional struggles?***

Whether this is in an effort to truly improve the health and nutritional status of an individual, or to capitalize on the vulnerability of those with diet-related chronic diseases to purchase their new *"Keto"* book or diet plan—any change in diet demands a background of evidence-based nutritional science, which should be accessible and translated to help the public's autonomy in making nutritionally sounds choices.

You've likely heard a few of the following statements about low-carbohydrate diets:

1) Insulin is the fat storage hormone.

2) Carbohydrates cause huge spikes in insulin, leading to weight-gain.

3) Eating a low-carbohydrate diet activates our satiety signals and hormones, making us eat less.

4) A low-carbohydrate diet can reverse type II diabetes.

5) Nutritional authorities, dietitians and doctors reject a low-carbohydrate diet due to industry pressures.

The issue with these statements is that they don't tell the entire story and are more mythical than factual. When deciding if a low-carbohydrate diet is right for you, it's not as black and white as it may appear as **everyone's metabolism, insulin sensitivity and gene expression is different**. This increases in complexity when applying these diets within the context of chronic diseases, including obesity and diabetes.

Let's break down each of these myths and discuss the current nutrition science behind them.

Myth #1: Insulin is the fat storage hormone

Insulin is a hormone that is released from our pancreas during the "fed" state, or when the nutrients from a meal are broken down and released into our bloodstream to be used by our body. Insulin acts as a "key" to unlock insulin-dependent organs access to the glucose in our bloodstream, namely the heart, fat tissue and muscles.

Insulin is released when there is not only a rise of glucose (from carbohydrates) in our blood stream, **but also when there is a rise in**

amino acids (from protein). Many advocates preaching the low carb/anti-insulin narrative often conveniently ignore or are not aware of this fact.

Once glucose or amino acids enter the cell thanks to insulin, the body has its own priorities to meet other than simply storing fat. This includes stimulating ATP production for the cell, anabolic protein and glycogen synthesis and restoring our blood sugar and amino acid concentrations back to baseline.

Fun Fact: Glycogen storage, found in our liver and our muscles, is evolutionarily speaking, a life-saving source of blood sugar (or energy). When faced with a fight-or-flight situation, adrenaline will elicit the breakdown of glycogen into glucose, providing us the energy to fight or flight the stressor.

If the needs of the cell are met, but there is an excess of energy which remains in the bloodstream (or in other words, if we consume too much energy for our body's needs) insulin will then facilitate the storage of fat into the adipose tissue. However, **this mechanism does not discriminate between the type of macronutrient which is found in excess within the diet.**

All macronutrients: fat, protein and carbohydrates are made out of carbon—which if present in excess, can be rearranged into a triglyceride to be stored in our fat tissue and consequently lead to weight-gain.

Therefore, it is not only carbohydrates, but it could also be an excess fat or protein leading to weight-gain and fat storage.

Myth #2: Carbohydrates cause huge spikes in insulin, leading to weight-gain

In a healthy individual, our levels of insulin in circulation remains within a healthy range even after consuming a meal high in carbohydrates. For the most part, as long as an individual has a healthy body weight, insulin spikes are kept within a normal, healthy range which is not conducive to weight-gain.

However, the difference in insulin levels varies greatly in a healthy individual compared to someone with insulin-resistance.

How does insulin-resistance occur? It's not directly from the over-consumption of sugar, but from the presence of excess body weight. Any excess of fat tissue contributes to inflammation, and the fat deposits around our organs interferes with insulin-signalling. In this case, insulin levels are chronically higher at all times because the body is working harder to make sure blood sugar levels return to normal.

Insulin does facilitate fat storage *in the presence of excess energy intake*, and it also inhibits the breakdown of fat. This ultimately creates an environment conducive to weight-gain **in an individual with insulin resistance.** This is the overarching rationale in prescribing a low-carbohydrate diet for those with insulin resistance.

What can improve insulin-resistance? **The opposite of what causes it.**

Weight-loss improves insulin resistance. A recent randomized controlled trial points to similar weight-loss between those who followed a high-quality low-carb and high-carb diet. Rather than pointing to a certain macronutrient causing weight-loss, the common denominator between these diets is that they were consumed at an *energy deficit, causing weight-loss and improving insulin signalling.*

Myth #3: Eating a low-carbohydrate diet activates our satiety signals and hormones, making us eat less

When a diet is low in carbohydrates, it means that the proportion of calories increase from fat and protein. These macronutrients are considered to increase satiety, therefore reducing overall energy intake and leading to weight-loss.

This part is true. I'm sure we have all experienced the satiety advantages of having a breakfast that included fats and protein (such as eggs, bacon, avocado, peanut butter) compared to one mostly comprised of carbohydrates (white toast, jam, sugary cereal). However, the determinants of satiety are much more complex than simply the macronutrient composition of the diet.

One of the most overlooked items in inducing satiety, *is the hormone insulin itself.* This is one of the primary hormones that feed back to our appetite-control centre in our brain to decrease our appetite. Our body is smart, as insulin is released when we are in the "fed" state, functioning to tell our brain that we don't need any more nutrients from diet and decreases our appetite. This is one snapshot into our body's complex homeostatic appetite-control mechanisms.

But, if insulin really decreases appetite, why do we experience less satiety after consuming a processed high-carbohydrate breakfas*t* (think white bread, sugary cereals) compared to a low-carb, high-fat, high protein breakfast (think bacon, eggs, avocado, peanut butter)?

To answer this question, we have to remember an important overarching theme in nutritional science: **No food, or macronutrient is ever consumed in isolation.** Therefore, we cannot condense our bodies complex response to food by blaming any single macronutrient.

A high fat/high protein breakfast sustains appetite as studies find that it increases the satiety hormone peptide PPY while decreasing the hunger hormone ghrelin. However, a high-protein breakfast will also elicit a release of insulin, which will also decrease hunger within our homeostatic pathway.

No one is recommending a refined high-carbohydrate breakfast, and it would never be a nutritionally optimal choice for breakfast. But this doesn't mean the answer is to immediately to go low-carb and only eat bacon and eggs for breakfast.

For example, we could easily enjoy a bowl of oatmeal with peanut butter and fruit.

While higher carbohydrate, the protein and fat content of such a breakfast is not to be overlooked: One cup of oats, with one cup milk and one tablespoon of peanut butter would yield about 18 g of fat and 22 g of protein, allowing us to reap the satiety inducing benefits of fat and protein without sacrificing carbohydrates.

Myth #4: A low-carbohydrate diet is the only diet that can reverse type II diabetes

In type II diabetes, the body is less responsive to the hormone insulin, resulting in a build-up of sugar in the bloodstream. As previously discussed, the most common cause of insulin resistance is excessive body weight, where fat deposits around organs decrease the effectiveness of insulin.

The build-up of sugar in the bloodstream over time can cause serious health problems, including vision damage, nerve damage, heart and kidney disease. As sugar is found in the bloodstream, many people are quick to think that a low-carbohydrate, or low sugar diet is the best, or only way to reverse type II diabetes.

While it is possible to follow a low-carbohydrate diet to improve blood sugar levels in those living with type II diabetes, it is not the only way to manage the disease. For example, the best way to improve **insulin signalling is if weight-loss is achieved. Weight loss** can be achieved on a diet of varying macronutrient compositions, including those that are higher in carbohydrates. The best diet for weight-loss is the one that you can stick with, and for some this may be a lower-carb diet, for others it is one that includes complex carbohydrates.

It's also important to highlight a few potential risks of following a low carbohydrate diet in the context of type II diabetes. In the case of poorly controlled diabetes, improper insulin signalling will produce ketone bodies to serve as an alternative source of fuel in the blood stream. The level of ketone bodies will only increase while following a low carbohydrate diet, increasing the risk of ketoacidosis. Ketoacidosis is a rare, but serious condition in those living with diabetes where the blood becomes too acidic and requires immediate medical attention.

Another risk with following a low carbohydrate diet is that fat intake will increase. While monounsaturated and polyunsaturated fats are great for health, replacing carbohydrates with saturated or trans-fats can increase the risk of heart disease. As those living with diabetes are already at a higher risk of heart disease, they should be followed closely by their doctor and dietitian if deciding to follow a low carbohydrate diet.

Myth #5: Nutritional authorities, doctors and dietitians are lying to us

This is where it is important to emphasize the key differences between public health messaging and individualized nutritional interventions.

On a population level, there is simply not enough evidence to support a low-carbohydrate diet as a model diet for a healthy individual, or as a keystone nutritional intervention for chronic-diseases.

However, on an individual level, following a low carbohydrate diet may help you reach your goals. Working with a dietitian can help design a diet based on your unique health and nutritional needs, making sure the diet is safe, effective and sustainable.

As with all science, people need to be skeptical. A historic lesson in nutritional skepticism is when <u>The Sugar Institute funded-studies to blame fat instead of refined carbohydrates on coronary artery disease</u> in the 1950's and 1960's, which had a tremendous influence on our nutritional landscape. However, there has also been <u>lobbying from the Meat and Dairy industry</u> to have their own food-group in National Food Guides in efforts to promote the agricultural sector.

Overzealous nutritional advice must be taken with a grain of salt and perceived through a lens of skepticism. Remember that the one to come up with the new, exciting and promising diet to reverse anything, is also the one to make the most money.

Furthermore, many diets which are based off one certain macronutrient often completely dismiss the complexity of food, nutrition, the psyche and the human being. Remember, not one certain food, or macronutrient is consumed in isolation.

If anything, **the rise of obesity is not because we stopped consuming a low-carbohydrate diet.** If speaking exclusively diet-wise, the rise of obesity is more likely due to the overconsumption of cheap, readily available processed foods: which encompass carbohydrates, protein and fats, alike.

Vegan & Vegetarian Diets

If you've ever visited Reddit, you are likely familiar with the lively discussions about nearly any topic, providing great advice and suggestions from real people. In fact, Reddit can be extremely useful for learning about vegan and vegetarian diets, especially for different ingredient substitutions, yummy recipes and other quick tips and tricks for those following a plant-based diet.

However, some discussion that crosses these forums is concerning from a nutritional standpoint. For example, one user recommended that a diet comprised of potatoes, legumes and bread would be sufficient to meet protein needs. Another suggested to purchase expensive plant-based protein powders to maximize their *"fat-burning"* potential. Others explained that plant-based diets are absolutely the most affordable option for those struggling to make ends meet.

While many of these off-hand comments are relatively harmless, the cumulation of individual suggestions can make nutrition seem even more confusing than it already is.

In the democratization of information, nutrition has been hit hard with wide-spread misinformation and misinterpretation. Therefore, the purpose of this chapter on vegan and vegetarian diets is to provide more **context** to the world of plant-based diets, so that you can be empowered to make better decisions about your health, well-being and nutrition.

Myth #1: Plant-based = vegan and vegetarian diets

The truth is that there is no official definition as to what a plant-based diet is. If the mention of plant-based diets conjures up images of birdseed, granola and huge green smoothies, you've likely been influenced by Instagram influencers.

The key with plant-based diets is right in its name, **plant-based — not plants only.** This means that almost anyone, regardless of preferred dietary patterns (*vegetarian, pescatarian, omnivore, paleo, keto or whatever*) can adopt a plant-based diet.

When eating plant-based, the main focus is placed on the majority of your plate (or bowl) being plant-foods. This can include making half your plate vegetables and having a combination of fruit/protein for snacks. It's little additions like these which can make the totality of our diet more healthful, without adhering to a restrictive dietary pattern.

Myth #2: Plant-based diets are cheaper

Many individuals advocate for plant-based diets based on affordability. This does hold some merit, as fruits and vegetables can be purchased frozen or canned, and grains, nuts, legumes and seeds can be purchased dried or in bulk. However, it ultimately depends on an individual's physical and financial accessibility to these foods.

For some, purchasing an energy-dense fast-food meal for $4–5 dollars will be more cost and time efficient for a low-income individual who lives in a food desert. For time and resource-strapped families, purchasing bulk frozen grilled chicken strips may be a more financially savvy way to ensure their children meet their protein needs.

Plant-based diets demand a certain level of food and cooking literacy, time, and effort. Furthermore, the cost of fruits and vegetables experienced an increase in 2020 and well into 2021.

Is this an excuse to forego all efforts to eat healthy? Absolutely not, but plant-based diets may not be a valid recommendation for universal health and wellbeing, as it disregards important socioeconomic determinants of health.

Myth #3: You need to combine plant-proteins to get a complete protein

This old-age myth comes from the idea that plant-proteins lack a certain amino acid, which means that combining foods will make sure no amino acids fall through the cracks.

However, the words "complete" protein is misleading, as all plant-foods contain a complete amino acid profile. The difference lies in the *amount* of essential amino acids per source of plant-based food which determine the quality of the protein source.

Some sources of plant-proteins are better than others. For example, tofu and quinoa are considered the highest quality plant-based protein sources due to their amino acid availability. The best rule of thumb is to ensure that you are eating a **variety of foods** each day to meet your protein requirement.

Myth #4: On a vegetarian or vegan plant-based diet, you don't need to supplement

Many advocates for vegetarian and vegan diets claim that you can meet all your micronutrient needs without supplementation. Unlike protein, vitamins and minerals demand a bit more attention to detail. If your plant-based diet excludes animal products, a few nutrients of concern include the following:

- **Vitamin B12:** You cannot find the same bioavailability of B12 in plants and often fortified foods such as soy milk and nutritional yeast may not be reliable (especially if you don't consume them every day and nutritional content differs by manufacturer). Supplement Vitamin B12 with around <u>100–150 mcg</u> per day.
- **Vitamin D:** Vitamin D is rarely found naturally in foods, and synthesis of Vitamin D within your skin is unreliable year-round, especially if you live in a seasonal climate. Supplement with around <u>1000 IU</u> per day.
- **Iron:** While you can find iron in plant foods, it is less bioavailable in its non-heme form. You can meet your iron requirements by regularly consuming lentils, fortified cereals and grain products, pumpkin seeds and some nut butters.

Myth #5: Plant-based diets are the healthiest dietary pattern for everyone

Plant-based diets are certainly a healthy dietary pattern, however given the above they are not always realistic, or helpful, for every single individual as our relationship with food extends beyond what's on our plate.

Take for example an individual with chronic kidney disease, where their protein, phosphate and potassium intake must be limited to avoid progressing their disease state. In this instance, an entirely plant-based diet (*high in potassium and phosphate*) is not always the overarching recommendation.

Similarly, people living with obesity or those living in low-income neighbourhoods with limited access to healthy foods — prescribing "*plant-based diets*" are unlikely to solve the root of their health problems.

The Bottom Line

Going back to the well-intended users on the reddit forum; a plant-based diet is unlikely the be-all and end-all answer to everyone's problems. And there are several misconceptions around what it means to eat plant-based in the first place.

It is undeniable that most individuals would benefit from adding more whole foods, including vegetables, fruits, legumes, grains, nuts & seeds into their diet. Plant-based diets even have pretty robust science behind them to prove their impacts on improving cardiovascular disease, diabetes and even cancer risks.

The most important takeaway from this article is that we should find a way of eating **which is sustainable to us.** Good nutrition shouldn't focus on the singularity of one macronutrient over another, but should consider our nutritional goals, lifestyle, cooking skills, current disease management and quality of life as a whole

---

With more time on their hands over the past year, individuals flocked to the grocery stores and began to cook more for themselves and try new foods. This resulted in the discovery of many new food trends and foods on the market. In this chapter, we will cover two of the trendiest foods in 2021: the rise of oat milk and a new gluten-free flour, banana flour.

Food Trend #1: The Art & Science Behind Oat Milk

Swedish Scientist Rickard Oste first created oat milk in the early 1990's. He was a food scientist studying lactose intolerance. He wanted to create an environmentally friendly drink which contained no lactose sugar. Ahead of his time, he created a thick, creamy product with natural sweetness thanks to the natural sugars found in oats.

Oat milk naturally contains more starch than soy, almond or rice milk where dairy milk has no starch. Enzymes are added to the oat milk mixture which allows for the release of natural sugar molecules from the starch, which is why oat milk has naturally sweet, nutty taste.

Oat milk significantly decreases greenhouse gas emissions and intensive water usage compared to levels required dairy farming. For example, one litre of dairy milk is estimated to take of 1000 litres of water to produce, while one litre of oat milk only requires around 48 litres of water to produce.

It is important to note that these numbers are not 100% reflective of the intensity of resources required to create oat or dairy milk. For example, rainwater counts towards the water required for crops and paddock.

The Nutritional Science Behind Oat Milk

Unfortunately, drinking one cup of oat milk is not comparable to eating a bowl of oatmeal. However, oat milk still has some notable health benefits and deserves to be compared with other milks and milk alternatives.

Oat milk might help lower LDL-cholesterol levels

Oat milk contains β-glucan, a type of soluble fibre which is proven to reduce LDL-cholesterol levels. β-glucan is a non-starch carbohydrate, which forms complexes with the cholesterol containing bile-salts in our intestine.

One study showed that diets supplemented with around 3g of β-glucan decreased LDL-cholesterol levels by 5–7% compared to control diets.

One cup of oat milk is estimated to contain around 1.3 grams of β-glucans, whereas one-cup of oats contains closer to 3 g. Oat milk might help you up your β-glucan intake without having to consume copious amounts of oats.

Oat milk is lower in sugar, and lactose-free

Non-dairy milks get a bad rap on their sugar content, however many people fail to realize that dairy milks have a significant amount of naturally occurring sugar, mostly in the form of the disaccharide **lactose**.

For comparison, one cup of 1% dairy milk has 12–13 g of naturally occurring sugar, while one cup of unsweetened oat milk contains only 6 grams of naturally occurring sugar from the oats and contains no lactose.

This is especially beneficial for those who are lactose intolerant. Nearly half of the adult-population in North America is

<u>lactose-intolerant</u> as the function of our lactase enzyme, lactase, significantly decreases after being weaned off breastmilk.

Oat milk is lower in protein

Oat milk has significantly less protein, at only 4 g per cup compared to 8 g found in one cup of cow's milk. However, this is higher than all other non-dairy alternatives except for soy milk. Soy milk remains the non-dairy alternative, which is on par with cow's milk, which contains 8 g of protein per cup.

While oat milk is safe for children and teens, it shouldn't replace soy or cow's milk if it is relied on as a source of protein. As with all milks, oat milk should **never** replace breastmilk or infant formula.

Oat milk is a good source of calcium and vitamin D (most of the time)

Commercial manufacturers will fortify the milk with calcium, vitamin D and B12 to make it comparable to dairy milk and other non-dairy milks. While it varies amongst brands, in general one cup of oat milk will provide <u>at least 30–50% daily value of calcium, vitamin D and B12.</u>

But, fortification of these milks is not always required by law depending on where you live. Always make sure to read the nutrition facts label and shake your milk carton before pouring! Nutrients often settle to the bottom of the carton.

Note that with homemade oat-milks will not have vitamin D, B12 or calcium as you can't simply fortify milk in your kitchen. If you plan on making homemade oat milk, make sure plan on getting these nutrients from other sources.

The world of alternative flours appears to be expanding each week. From rice, coconut, buckwheat, sorghum to everything in between, there is definitely no shortage of different flours to choose from.

Whether it's for an individual living with celiac disease who is looking for a gluten-free alternative or a food scientist looking for a shelf-stable ingredient, the differing nutrition profile of these flours can help increase the diversity, and creativity of the foods available to us.

The newest addition to this roster? Enter **banana flour,** a tropical flour which has notable health, environmental and food processing benefits, and might just be the next big thing in the world of flours.

What exactly is banana flour, and how is it made?

Banana flour is made from dehydrating and grinding underripe **green bananas.** The flour originated regions in Africa and Jamaica as an innovative, cheaper alternative to traditional wheat flours.

On average, it takes 10 kg of underripe green bananas to make 1 kg of banana flour. While these processing losses are significantly higher than wheat flour, where 1kg of wheat can produce about 950 g of flour, the environmental impact may be offset by the ability to repurpose underripe bananas which would normally be crop losses.

For example, the demand for banana flour could help farmers recoup otherwise lost earnings from underripe bananas, which are often refused by suppliers and grocery stores.

What is the nutritional science and the health benefits behind banana flour?

1. Banana flour is rich in resistant starch which helps promote a healthy gut microbiome

What distinguishes banana flour from other alternative flours, such a rice, oat, tapioca or potato is its **resistant starch content.** Resistant starch a type of prebiotic, meaning it acts as food for the trillions of microorganisms which reside in our gut microbiome. Compared to ripe bananas, which have 1–15% resistant starch content, banana flour provides up to 70% resistant starch content.

With the rise of processed foods, our consumption of prebiotics, including resistant starch has decreased dramatically. This runs parallel to the fact that over 70% of Canadians do not meet the recommended servings of fruits and vegetables, where many fruits & vegetables including mushrooms, artichokes, asparagus and apples (to name a few) are **natural sources of prebiotics.**

Diet is a large modulator of the gut microbiome, and heavily processed diets are associated with disrupting the gut microbiome, otherwise known as "dysbiosis".

Prebiotics, including resistant starches, are important for our gut microbiome because of their ability to stimulate the growth of beneficial microorganisms. These microorganisms will ferment the resistant starch into short-chain fatty acids. Multiple studies have reported the health benefits of these short-chain fatty acids in improving digestive health as they act as fuel for the cells which line our gastrointestinal tract. Emerging evidence also suspects that a heathy gut microbiome plays a role in preventing obesity, diabetes, depression and several other diseases.

However, the exact health benefits, or short-falls, of the gut microbiome & it's relationship to diet is extremely difficult to pin-point difficult because everyone's gut microbiome different. In fact, each individual's microbiome can vary as much as <u>80–90%,</u> as such clinicians and scientists cannot agree on a universal definition of what a healthy gut microbiome is.

2. Banana flour has a lower glycemic index

Banana flour has a lower-glycemic index compared to other flours, such as wheat, oat, tapioca, rice and potato due to its high resistant starch content. A lower glycemic index means that there is a slower release of glucose (a type of sugar) into the bloodstream, resulting in a slower rise in the hormone insulin. Slower releases of insulin are associated with increased satiety and decreased weight gain.

However, it should be noted that when banana flour is used in **baking at temperatures <u>above 140F</u>**, the heat will cause it to lose some of its resistant starch content as it is converted into digestible sugars. This means that the low-glycemic index along with its prebiotic properties are unlikely to be maintained after baking.

3. Banana flour is a rich source of potassium

Banana flour, like bananas, are very rich source of **potassium.** 35 g of banana flour has around <u>300 mg of potassium</u>, the same amount which is found in a medium-sized banana. **Potassium** plays an important role in heart health, especially when it comes to maintaining healthy blood pressure.

It is estimated that 1 in 4 Canadians live with hypertension, or <u>high blood pressure</u>. High blood pressure increases the risk of heart disease, strokes and kidney failure and is attributed to the excess amount of **sodium** consumed in the diet.

Potassium plays an interesting role in decreasing blood pressure by counteracting the effects of sodium. In fact, consuming foods higher in potassium is <u>more effective</u> in reducing high blood pressure than decreasing sodium intake alone.

While the most realistic way of increasing your potassium intake may not be through eating cookies and muffins made with banana flour, try adding a spoonful of banana flour to oatmeal or smoothies.

4. Banana flour is naturally gluten-free

As banana flour is made simply from bananas, it is a naturally **gluten-free flour**. This means that they are suitable flours for those living with celiac disease or have diagnosed sensitivities to gluten. Gluten is a protein found in wheat which is responsible for the important for rising and integrity of baked goods.

If used in baking, banana flour is a great gluten-free flour substitute in baking *denser* goods such as breads, cookies, pancakes and muffins. Banana flour does not require any additional binders such as with other gluten-free flours. The general rule of thumb is to substitute 1 cup of wheat flour with ¾ cup banana flour.

What's the bottom line?

Banana flour certainly has many potential health benefits and is a flour that can be enjoyed by those who need to avoid gluten. When consumed raw, it is a rich source of resistant starch. It is also a rich source of potassium and has a low-glycemic index.

However, it's important to remember that **these health benefits *are not mutually exclusive to banana flour*** and can be found in plenty of other affordable and more readily accessible foods, including fresh fruits & vegetables.

That being said, banana flour certainly remains a creative, new flour that has many attractive food processing and nutritional benefits. Don't be surprised if you see banana flour as an up-and-coming superfood in the next few months, and if you do you will already be ahead of the trend—armed with the knowledge of the scientific genius behind this flour.

Chapter 8: Food Security & Socioeconomic Determinants of Nutrition

Throughout this book, we have discussed many things about nutrition and health. From the basic macronutrients, to sports nutrition, digestive & mental health and even the debate between low carbohydrate and high carbohydrate diets, all these topics make one big assumption: **That we have the financial and physical access to foods.**

While it may seem simple at first, let's dig a bit deeper to truly understand what this means.

When we think of having good nutritional status, we often think of healthy weight, normal blood pressure, no overt nutrient deficiencies or other metabolic complications. All of these are important, however are often the end-product of cumulative behaviours and our social and physical environments, which run much deeper than simply the foods we eat.

Besides being able to obtain healthy foods, eat an overall balanced diet, and get adequate physical activity, it all leads to a bigger question: *what else could be hindering an individual to take ownership of their nutritional status, and achieve and maintain health?*

Perhaps one answer lies within our environment and our education. When we critique an adult's ability to access nutritious foods, their ability to be skeptical about food and wellness marketing and their health status, we should consider their nutrition education.

We live in a world where every cent count, and we want to make sure the cents available to spend on foods provide us good nutrition in return. For example, **Canadians are often encouraged to spend only 10–15% of their income on groceries.**

Fun Fact: In most countries, including Canada, the poverty line is measured by something known as a "basket measure". You can think of the basket measure as a real basket, filled with the basic, but required items (including food) or services which cost money to live a modest life. If you can't afford these items in your basket, you are living below the poverty line.

In Canada, the lowest basket measure is about $17,000 per one individual, per year. Based on the recommended 10–15% of income to be put towards groceries, this leaves individuals between roughly 30–45$ per week to be spent on groceries.

How could $45 be translated into providing nutritionally adequate, delicious and culturally appropriate foods on the table?

It's not easy. (And remember many people are living below the poverty line, and likely have *much less* than $45).

Grocery shopping on a limited budget presents a sufficient challenge, and the issue deepens in complexity for those with limited nutritional education and food preparation skills.

Unfortunately, nutrition education is extremely limited. The backbone of nutrition education to children and teens cannot continue to solely consist of calories in, and calories out—or the infamous *"how many cubes of sugar in your soft drink?"*. These activities are not providing the tangible skills needed to truly benefit one's ability to take ownership of their nutritional status.

Nutrition education can provide one with confidence in making nutritionally sound and balanced food choices while remaining within budget. Knowing different kinds of plant-proteins to pair to make complete proteins, choosing fruits and vegetables in season, and choosing less processed options can do wonders both budget and nutrition-wise.

Food preparation skills will cover the basics once these affordable foods are brought home. Understanding simple preparation skills such as chopping vegetables and making a simple dressing or cooking rice on the stove not only puts food on the table, but also serves as a life-long skill that improves health, wellbeing and sense of independence.

However, these skills cannot be taught in isolation, and it is common for those from low-income households to demonstrate more resourcefulness with their budget and grocery shopping than those of higher income households. But—if we can empower people to take ownership of their nutrition, as well as prioritize it at a healthy-age **we know being able to make healthy meals goes beyond just good nutrition**. Perhaps nutrition education will be able to bring people together, foster a sense of independence, and might event improve mental health.

However, our systematic lack of proper nutrition education and food preparation skills are not making healthy eating a default option. Rather, the availability of cheap processed foods makes many people more likely to adapt these diets instead.

Energy-rich, nutrient poor diets contribute to what's known as the "*double-burden*" of malnutrition, defined as the co-existence of obesity and nutrient deficiencies. We also know that chronic excessive energy intake can result in abdominal obesity, insulin resistance, hypertension and dyslipidemia. These are risk factors for diet-related chronic diseases including cardiovascular disease and type II diabetes (this is also known as *metabolic syndrome*).

For those who think in numbers, the issue of malnutrition is also reflected on an economic level. Published in 2018, "***The economic burden of not meeting food recommendations***" study estimates diet-related diseases to cost the Canadian Health Care System $13.8 billion per year.

But we know that transitioning from a processed, nutrient-poor diet for one rich in fresh fruits and vegetables, whole grains, and quality proteins is not as easy as it seems. And it's a privilege in itself to have the time, necessary kitchen equipment and access to groceries stores.

It's less on the fault of the individual, and more of the collective when we consider those who are experiencing any degree of food insecurity. Ultimately, we need to critique our nations collective nutritional status through the lens of our social infrastructure:

What are we doing to harness individuals, and in particularly today's youth, to take charge of their nutrition?

The next time we see someone in a poor nutritional status, instead of having them spearhead the blame, let's check our own privilege and ask ourselves:

- *Are we advocating for comprehensive and mandatory nutrition education in schools?*
- *Are we supporting community food programs and local food banks?*
- *Are we reducing food waste, or diverting food waste to those who could benefit?*
- *Are we making nutritional information accessible, and understandable, to the public?*

It's undeniable that we need to change the way we approach nutrition in today's society. However, in highlighting our lack of nutrition education simultaneously provides us with a potential solution:

Using nutrition education to blunt the impact of financial and physical barriers in accessing foods, while creating a useful tool to help people take ownership of their nutritional status.

Nutritional Privilege and Access to Food

The **ability to choose what you eat, and how often, is a huge privilege, and** the truth is that many people don't have control over the next meal that they will have.

They don't get to pour over the nutritional value of one food over another, enjoy their favourite dish at a trendy restaurant, or meander to their local farmers market to purchase in-season produce. They don't get to spend their Saturday's at Whole Foods, deciding between which alkaline, gluten-free, non-GMO food is best for their new keto diet.

In fact, many things often associated with good nutritional status, such as gaining weight, losing weight, avoiding, or overcoming a nutritional deficiency comes with a certain flavour of privilege.

Nutritional privilege can be dissected into one's physical and financial access to safe, nutritious and culturally appropriate foods. This is highly related to one's food security, defined by the Food and Agriculture Organization (FAO) as the ***secure access to sufficient amounts of safe and nutritious food for normal growth and development and an active and healthy life***.

When we have food security, we can most easily obtain good nutrition and we can appreciate our nutritional privilege. But what about others who aren't so lucky?

The strongest predictor of food security has historically been income. In Canada, the primary source of income for those with household food insecurity is **wages and salaries** not welfare or social assistance, contrary to popular belief. People living with food insecurity are working, but their means cannot extend into providing a sufficient amount of food for themselves or their families- a job is no longer enough.

The most alarming cases of food insecurity exist in Canada exists in the North. Food insecurity amongst Indigenous peoples in Nunavut is the most alarming, where 46% of all households are living with moderate or severe food insecurity. This is drastically inflated compared to the rest of Canada, where the national average is typically around 10–12%.

Food insecurity is an example of a real nutritional problem in Canada, where the reasoning for these problems delves deep into personal and collective determinants of health. The complex determinants of health which are rooted in this issue extend beyond the purpose of this chapter, bit it's important to highlight one population that **absolutely needs nutrition for change**. And efforts such as building healthy public policy, food subsidies, community and urban agriculture programs could have a real, sustainable impact on the health of this population.

For the nutritionally privileged, perceptions of "*good nutrition*" have deepened in complexity and extend beyond the simple definition provided by FAO above. On the other side of the spectrum, nutrition is now entrenched within the diet, wellness and food-industry, driving an overwhelming and undesirable industry response.

All of a sudden, we can't just eat fruits and vegetables, but only a certain kind, in a certain shape and colour. Our shopping cart isn't considered healthy unless we see labels displaying "*gluten-free*", "*non-GMO*", "*alkaline*" or other meaningless, nutritional jargon. These products are also alarmingly more expensive, further reserving the fulfillment of a constructed ideal of "*good nutrition*" for the financially privileged.

We also might preach certain diets, such as vegan or vegetarian as being the gate-keepers of good health and reserved for the environmental elite—without considering country foods (e.g. caribou, fish, elk) that <u>Indigenous people have skillfully and sustainably sourced in harmony with their ecosystem and environment.</u>

The wellness industry further capitalizes on our short-attention span, our endless pursuit of achieving "*health*" in combination with our limited and easily impressionable nutrition education. We are consequently sampled amongst an endless array of nutrition products and diets; when low-fat went out of trend, we went organic, gluten-free, keto, non-GMO, and even farm-to-table.

The profit-driven food and marketing industries are beyond skill-full in skewing our perception of how we equate nutrition to health. Food begins to be tied to self-actualization rather than a simple, inherent physiological requirement.

People living with food insecurity have notably less sovereignty over their own nutritional status. When living with less financial and physical access to healthful foods, they simply don't get to choose how their next meal may look like. If depending on the Food Bank, food hampers and baskets are sometimes nutritionally unbalanced, which in turn provides families no choice of feeding only refined carbohydrates for breakfast, lunch and dinner.

When convenience stores and fast-food restaurants are the only accessible means to obtain foods—or in other words, for people who are living in what is known as a food desert—it's a matter of survival to rely on these processed foods to quickly feed their family. These kinds of diets, while essential within the context provided, will unveil consequences when consumed over a lifetime. These low-nutrient high calorie foods contribute to what is known as the double-burden of malnutrition: ***the co-existence of nutrient deficiencies while being overweight or obese.***

This social issue deepens in complexity when those with less means are then blamed for their nutritional status—*"Only if you ate more fresh fruits and vegetables ..."* says the nutritionally privileged, while sipping their $7.99 collagen green smoothie *"... then you could be healthier, it's that easy!"*.

The other discourse we hear for this population is that they should just *"budget-better"* to improve their health and resolve food insecurity. The truth is that <u>those in low-income populations demonstrate highly resourceful skills</u>, and if armed with the right access to foods (i.e. not living in a food desert) they are more likely to purchase more nutrients per dollar compared to their higher earning counter-parts.

Now, we know that we have a real issue concerning nutrition and food security on our hands. We have people who cannot afford to eat, co-existing in an environment where over <u>63% of perfectly-edible foods are wasted.</u> We want change, and now more and more consumers are becoming aware of the issue—demanding low waste alternatives, compost and more local-foods.

But is the nutrition help really getting to where it needs to be?

While noble in intent, the issue arises when the diet, wellness and food industry begin to commercialize these well-intended demands. Instead of making way for community food programs, shared gardens and affordable grocery stores—tackling the real issue of food insecurity—the market provides us with natural, zero-waste and eco-friendly food stores. What comes with is are astronomical prices to pinch profits from the new wave of the *"privileged eco-conscious"* consumers. All of a sudden, only those who are financially comfortable can make the environmentally sound choice of arranging their bulk nuts and seeds in mason jars on the counter.

We have people who cannot afford to eat, co-existing in an environment where over 63% of perfectly edible foods are wasted.

The rise of the zero-waste, minimally processed foods and wellness products coincides with those living in increased rates of food insecurity. While those with privilege are feeding their self-actualization; refusing a plastic-straw, eating a $14 farm-to-table salad for lunch and purchasing over-priced bulk soba-noodles—there are people around the corner, existing within the same city, who cannot even put food on the table.

In fact, the Farm-to-Table movement initially began to connect low-income individuals with local farmers who needed a market for their produce. This helped strengthen communities and foster environmental responsibility all while working to close the gap of food insecurity. Likewise, it also drove the demand for large chain supermarkets to increase the number of suppliers from small and local farmers. I see win-wins here—as access to socially and environmentally responsible food choices should never be discriminated by economical slotting.

But the answer to solving true nutritional problems, such as food insecurity, and health inequalities goes beyond eating an optimal macronutrient profile, the pricy eco-zero waste stores or ordering the next trendy food box.

If we are lucky enough to have nutritional privilege—we can redefine what good nutrition means to us. And we definitely cannot continue to blame the individual for their nutritional status; whether underweight, overweight or simply consuming processed foods. Remember—those living with food insecurity have incomes from wages and salaries and granted access, are beyond resourceful with their budget to purchase healthy foods.

Perhaps this leads us to question other societal gate keepers of good nutrition—*over-priced grocery stores, poor urban planning, and insufficient healthy public policy.*

Guide to Zero Food Waste Meal Prepping

As mentioned above, over <u>63% of perfectly-edible foods are wasted, and mostly at the household level.</u> This means that large corporations or grocery stores do not hold most of the blame for food waste, but the power rests in the hands of the consumers. In this chapter, we will go over some tangible strategies to decrease food waste at home and save money – notable, **meal prep**.

What's the first thing that comes to mind when you hear "meal prep"? For many, it often brings about images of towers of Tupperware with identical portions of generic looking foods. Usually a combination of chicken, rice and broccoli all under an unflattering Instagram filter. Subsequently, the hashtags #mealprepgoals and #gains usually trail such photos.

It's easy to forget the 1/2 kg of pre-cooked quinoa left in the fridge for a week, or the salad that has that lovely metallic taste by Tuesday. And let's not forget that *trying-to-not-feel-guilty-feeling* when we buy a $13 meal at the cafeteria knowing very well that we have edible, but tasteless and failed dish of meal prep in the fridge back home.

To combat this, let's talk about to a *meal prep cycle*.

A meal prep cycle extends beyond portioning a ridiculous amount of food each Sunday night, buying bento-boxes, flimsy black microwavable containers or making Instagram able mason jar salads (*if you really think mason jars are a good container for salads, you're stuck in 2014*).

Instead, a meal prep cycle—as reflected in the name—concerns the true cycle of your meals, from the grocery store, to your fridge, preparation, and finally, to consumption. Think of it as examining your personal mini food-supply chain. Identify the kinks, working them out, and then enjoying the benefits; namely in lower grocery bills, less time spent in the kitchen, and reduced food waste.

How can I meal prep cycle?

The key to meal prep cycling is that **you don't focus on preparing a huge amount of food at once.**

Instead, pick a few factors to improve on and you are more likely to create an environment where meal prepping doesn't seem so impossible after all.

Let's dig in.

1. Clean up your fridge

Start with your at-home inventory and storage by cleaning and organizing your fridge, which is the first step in your food supply chain.

When you have good fridge hygiene, you can take an accurate inventory of the foods you currently have, the foods you need to use up quickly, and the foods you need to buy. This avoids food spoilage and ensures you don't over-purchase foods you may already have.

Top fridge hygiene tips:

1. Conduct a "fridge-harvest": Put together a bowl of vegetables that are about to go bad and prioritize cooking them within the next few days. Try roasting them, or cooking them into a large batch of soup.
2. Downsize sauces and leftovers into smaller containers to free-up space.
3. Ensure the foods you have are stored properly. Some tips include:

   - Separate your ethylene producers from the ethylene sensitive. *(e.g. separate bananas and avocados from apples, potatoes and broccoli).*
   - Store vegetables prone to wilting (*spinach, kale, cucumbers, carrots etc.*) in a high-humidity crisper drawer. If your fridge doesn't have this setting, make sure they are stored with as little open-air contact as possible.
   - Store meats at the bottom of the fridge to avoid juices spilling down and contaminating other foods.

In your first stab at establishing fridge hygiene, allow yourself to dispose of some items if you truly believe that they will hold you back from achieving true fridge sovereignty. Use it as a learning opportunity to acknowledge the waste, then move onto avoiding food waste in the future.

Eventually, you can start to apply the same tactic to your pantry and freezer, however the fridge is often the biggest culprit of food-waste in households, as it houses most perishable foods.

2. Make your grocery list and make it work double-duty.

After the storage and inventory is dealt with, it's time to place your order with your grocery list. But we want this grocery list to work for you, and not against you. Try the wrap or salad method to get two different meals out of the same ingredients.

Think of a group of ingredients, or flavours, that would go well in both a wrap and a salad and go from there. This step calls for some trial and error, some practice and creativity, but it is well worth it—especially if you're someone who gets bored of eating the same thing each day.

Some items that will work with the wrap and salad method include:

- Spinach, black beans, tomatoes, corn, salsa and tofu on rice (like a burrito bowl) or on a whole wheat wrap (like a burrito).

- Chickpeas, red onion, pickles, tahini, red pepper to make a chickpea salad, or to spread on toast.
- Sweet potato, coconut milk, red pepper, onion and tofu to make curry which could be served on rice, spinach or with naan.
- Home-made falafels with tomato, pickles, spinach, parsley, hummus and tahini on pitas. The same vegetables could be used to make a fattoush or tabbouleh salad.

Falafel wrap, where the same vegetables could be used to make a chickpea salad. (Photo by me).

Another method for starting out is to make a "building blocks" grocery list. This list will include a variety of fruits & vegetables, protein foods and whole grains to mismatch and make delicious meals throughout the week.

Once you decide on your meal strategy for the week, grab your list and remove everything thats already in your (newly organized) fridge, pantry and freezer. Then, with the help of a recipe, make sure to estimate your portion sizes and amounts needed for each item and head to the grocery store.

3. Cook it all up, all at once.

After your ordering (grocery shopping) step in your own personal supply chain is complete, the production stage—or preparation of foods is next up.

Try prepping in stages, rather than all at once.

- Cook all your vegetables. Roast them, boil them, fry them. And store them in a separate air-tight container in the fridge.
- Cook all your grains—rice, pasta, couscous, barley, quinoa (technically quinoa is a seed, but you get the point). Store it in an air-tight container in the fridge.
- Cook your vegetarian protein source: Baked tofu, crispy chickpeas, spiced-black beans, spinach falafels and store it in an air-tight container for a week.
- Other protein sources, such as eggs, fish and poultry — Prepare eggs the day of, and fish and poultry only 2–3 days in advance, maximum.

Now, take a look back at your fridge—you should have something lovely staring back at you: Prepped vegetables, grains and proteins ready for the week.

What is in your fridge, is what you must eat

Try to commit to eating these foods for the week and aim to have the least number of items left in your fridge as possible.

Most people fail in this area for several reasons.

Some people don't end up liking the food that they prepared; too bland, too salty, too spicy. This is normal and making tasty meals that last the week calls for some trial and error. Don't be discouraged if your first meal isn't a world-class delicacy—however, to avoid food waste, try these tips first to <u>save the flavour</u> if your first few attempts don't quite suite your palate.

Now, let's re-cap your supply chain

1. **Inventory & Storage**: Clean out your fridge, and store foods properly. Then, slowly start doing the same to your freezer and pantry.
2. **Ordering:** Make your grocery list, including amounts. Remember to make it work "double-duty" or with "building blocks" of food groups. Deduct what you already have on hand from this list.
3. **Production:** Prepare all your foods, all at once. Make sure to store them in proper, air-tight containers.
4. **Distribution:** Portion out your meals each-day, and ideally the night before into a Tupperware. Commit to finishing each of your prepped meals.

And repeat.

Remember, when starting out, **try improving just one factor** out of this list, rather than doing an entire cycle. Having a clean fridge will do wonders in reducing food spoilage, which can help you manage your meal prep.

When we critique our own food procurement habits, we are operating our own micro-level sustainable food system. Notably, we are tackling the issue of reducing waste at the household level— which accounts for an astonishing 63% of perfectly healthy foods suitable for human consumption wasted each year.

Tackling food waste is also consistent with the Sustainable Development Goals (SDGs), which outline the framework of the

United Nations ambitious, but possible, plan to create a Zero Hunger world by 2030.

Conclusion – Nutrition in 2021

The definition of good nutrition is multi-factorial and extends beyond the foods that are found directly on your plate. Nutrition must consider a multitude of different aspects, including food preferences, budget, allergies and food sensitivities, motivation to cook and even choosing who we want to eat with. In other words, **nutrition is highly individualized**, as it should be.

From a biological standpoint, we need macronutrients and micronutrients to survive, thrive and even fend off diseases. Nutrients don't just provide us with energy but regulate the physiological functions of our body down to the cellular level. Nutrition is impactful, and what we put into our bodies every day is transformational in how we function and perform each and every day. However, most evidence points towards consuming an **overall healthy dietary pattern**, including one that is rich in different fruits and vegetables, plant proteins, lean animal proteins, whole grains, nuts and seeds is **more effective** than focusing on a single nutrient.

But, from a real-life standpoint, the healthiest diet for us may be completely different from others. For those with food sensitivities, preferences or during special occasions, healthy eating can look very different. Eliminating gluten for one person may help resolve digestive issues, while it may decrease the quality of life for another. Following a low-carbohydrate diet might improve blood sugar levels for some people, while it could lead to nutrient deficiencies for others. Eating a slice of homemade cake at a gathering may reduce be more effective at reducing stress than supplementing with all the vitamins and minerals in the world. Remember, that the human relationship with food is not simply based on replenishing our nutrient and energy needs.

We hope that this book has armed you with the different nuances that exist in nutrition and will continue to exist throughout 2021. There are many different diets and foods that are best for different people, and the way you eat this year may be drastically different from the years before. Ultimately, we challenge you to take this information and think of **what good nutrition and healthy eating means to you, and not to others**. While there is no one optimal one-size fits approach to eating, there is certainly an approach that works for you. Let's make that a focus for 2021.